Social Work, Poverty and
Social Exclusion

Social Work, Poverty and Social Exclusion

Dave Backwith

Open University Press

Open University Press
McGraw-Hill Education
McGraw-Hill House
Shoppenhangers Road
Maidenhead
Berkshire
England
SL6 2QL

email: enquiries@openup.co.uk
world wide web: www.openup.co.uk

and Two Penn Plaza, New York, NY 10121-2289, USA

First published 2015

A catalogue record of this book is available from the British Library

ISBN-13: 978-0-335-24585-7
ISBN-10: 0-335-24585-4
eISBN: 978-0-335-24586-4

Library of Congress Cataloging-in-Publication Data
CIP data applied for

Typeset by Transforma Pvt. Ltd., Chennai, India

Fictitious names of companies, products, people, characters and/or data that may be used herein (in case studies or in examples) are not intended to represent any real individual, company, product or event.

Printed and bound by CPI Group (UK) Ltd, Croydon, CR0 4YY

Praise for this book

"Dave Backwith's new book should be required reading for every social work student, as well as by managers, policy makers and experienced practitioners. Carefully researched and reasoned, it challenges social work to overcome the danger of treating poverty as the inevitable backdrop to practice and to actively address the intimate, daily, damaging impact of poverty in most service users' lives. Throughout, using frequent telling case studies, Backwith confronts the complexities of practice and asks big questions about the political and policy context of social work."

Paul Bywaters, Professor of Social Work, Coventry University, UK

"Dave Backwith provides social work with a strong values-based argument for politically engaged practice to address poverty and social exclusion. He advocates for 'making space' to address poverty and social exclusion, with an approach that eschews individual and pathological responses, instead emphasising a community-based and collective/mutual aid orientation. The book is informed by ecological and health inequalities perspectives and with chapters on children and families, older people and mental health, should be essential reading for all social workers."

Kate Karban, Senior Lecturer in Social Work, University of Bradford, UK, Co-convenor, Social Work and Health Inequalities Network, 2010–2014

"This book provides a comprehensive review of theory, research and policy on poverty and social exclusion. It identifies the forces which have narrowed social work's responses to poor people, and how practice could become more generous and imaginative."

Bill Jordan, Professor of Social Work, Plymouth University, UK

"Dave Backwith has successfully argued that social workers need to practice with a full appreciation of the impact of poverty and social exclusion on the people who need their assistance. This is, as he argues, essential for all areas of social work. His book therefore represents essential reading for all connected to the delivery of social work, students, practitioners and managers alike."

Mark Lymbery, University of Nottingham, UK

Contents

List of 'What do you think?' exercises   ix
List of tables and figures   xi
List of abbreviations   xiii
Acknowledgements   xv

1   Introduction   1

2   Poverty and social work   11

3   Understanding social exclusion   32

4   Broken Britain? The social context of poverty and social exclusion   51

5   Children and families: poverty, abuse and practice   76

6   Old age: a new social divide?   97

7   Mental distress, recovery and mutual aid   115

8   Making space: tackling poverty and social exclusion   139

9   Conclusion: love in a cold climate   161

Appendix: Fair Access to Care Services (FACS) bandings   171

References   173

Index   187

List of 'What do you think?' exercises

1.1	What is poverty?	2
1.2	The experience of poverty and poverty awareness	8
2.1	The 'deserving' and 'undeserving' poor	12
2.2	Relative poverty and necessities	16
2.3	Reducing poverty: 'deserving' and 'undeserving' social groups?	19
2.4	'Getting organized': credit unions and agency	26
3.1	'The importance of blame'	34
3.2	The discourse of 'Troubled Families'	36
3.3	Disability and discourses of exclusion	47
4.1	The responsibility gap: transformation of communities?	53
4.2	Globalization and social work practice	55
4.3	Why do poor people die young?	57
4.4	Domestic violence, family poverty and children's health	61
4.5	Social work and health inequalities	65
4.6	Young women, social exclusion and group work	68
4.7	Parenting and poverty	70
5.1	Living with hardship: going without	78
5.2	Stigma and self-esteem: accessing services	84
5.3	Social exclusion: 2 to 3 per cent?	87
5.4	Domestic violence, family poverty and social exclusion	90
6.1	A demographic time bomb?	100
6.2	'Care and control': social inclusion without consent?	107
7.1	Mental distress and social exclusion	117
7.2	Conduct disorders	121
7.3	The 'toxic trio' and 'storing up' mental distress?	124
7.4	Why do ethnic inequalities in mental health persist?	130
8.1	The 'deserving' and 'undeserving' poor revisited	140
8.2	'Just do it', making space in adult services	148
8.3	CSW and social inclusion	151
8.4	Homelessness and sensory impairment	154
9.1	Family poverty: class and control	163
9.2	Authoritarian social work?	166

List of tables and figures

Tables

Table 1.1	Defining poverty	2
Table 1.2	'What does poverty mean to you?'	8
Table 2.1	'Deserving' and 'undeserving' cases	12
Table 2.2	Poverty index: necessities of modern life?	16
Table 2.3	Poverty index: changes in necessities	18
Table 2.4	Household incomes at 60 per cent HBAI poverty line 2010/11	18
Table 3.1	Three ways of asking about disability	48
Table 5.1	'Challenges of engagement': contrasting perspectives of professionals and hard to reach families	88
Table 6.1	Factors in social isolation and low social participation	106
Table 8.1	A comparison of traditional and community-orientated approaches to social work	153
Table 8.2	Types of needs assessment	156

Figures

Figure 2.1	Relative poverty by age group (%) 1996 to 2010	20
Figure 2.2	The cycle of deprivation	21
Figure 2.3	UK Poverty: 1979 to 2008/9	24
Figure 4.1	Cigarette smoking prevalence and deprivation in Great Britain, 1973 and 2004	59
Figure 5.1	Proportion (%) of parents in poor families who could not afford selected items	79
Figure 5.2	'Groups whose problems are multiple and overlapping can lead to social exclusion in later life'	86
Figure 5.3	The Common Assessment Framework	93
Figure 6.1	Social exclusion of older people: forms and likely characteristics	99

List of abbreviations

BASW	British Association of Social Workers
BME	black and minority ethnic
BPS	bio-psycho-social
CSW	community social work
COS	Charity Organization Society
DfE	Department for Education
DPM	Disabled People's Movement
DRE	delivering race equality
DSW	deviant social work
DWP	Department for Work and Pensions
IFSW	International Federation of Social Work
JRF	Joseph Rowntree Foundation
MUD	moral underclass discourse
ONS	Office for National Statistics
PCS	personal, cultural and structural
PIP	Personal Independence Payment
PSE	Poverty and Social Exclusion
RCVP	Riots, Communities and Victims Panel
RED	redistribution discourse
SCIE	Social Care Institute for Excellence
SETF	Social Exclusion Task Force
SEU	Social Exclusion Unit
SID	social intregration discourse
SSD	social services departments
SWAN	Social Work Action Network
SWP	social work practice
TTC	Time to Change
WCA	Work Capability Assessment
WHO	World Health Organization

Acknowledgements

The ideas in this book have been developed in discussions with student social workers, from whose insight and know-how I have benefited greatly.

Many 'frontline' social workers and managers helped with the research for this book. Their contribution has been vast and several people went 'above and beyond' in their efforts to assist me. As I am bound to preserve anonymity I cannot name them but would like to record my gratitude to these, invariably, busy people.

Several friends and colleagues have assisted me in different ways; in particular I would like to thank Ken Johnson, Paula Sobiechowska, Sue Harrington, Carol Munn-Giddings and Ros Hunt. When I was on the last lap Julie Scott's painstaking proof-reading was worth much more than chocolates can repay. Finally, I owe a special debt to Maire Maisch, without whose unwavering support and guidance this book would not have been written.

Acknowledgements

1 Introduction

> The most striking feature that clients of social services have in common is poverty and deprivation.
>
> (Schorr, 1992, quoted in Lymbery, 2001: 373)

As Schorr suggests, poverty, social exclusion and their consequences are near-universal characteristics of social work practice. For some service user groups the extent of deprivation is extreme. Care leavers, for example:

> . . . are more likely than young people who have not been in care to have poorer educational qualifications, lower levels of participation in post-16 education, be young parents, be homeless, and have higher levels of unemployment, offending behaviour and mental-health problems.
>
> (Stein, 2006: 273)

Similarly, the state enforced destitution of asylum seekers:

> . . . has led some individuals to self-harm and attempt suicide. Pregnant women and those with children cause particular concern. They often delay applying for support until late in pregnancy, and once they receive it are expected to live on vouchers for as little as £38 per week.
>
> (Refugee Council, 2006: 12–13)

Poverty and social exclusion are not only endemic, there is also a causal relationship which works in both directions: the issues which bring social workers into service users' lives are often caused or compounded by poverty and social exclusion and vice-versa. This is true, for example, of disability, mental distress and child abuse.

Despite this, there is a danger that poverty can become part of the background music of practice. In relation to older people, for example, Foster (2011: 348) warns that social workers might overlook poverty because, paradoxically, 'it is assumed that it is an inherent and integral feature of service users' lives'. While (Perry, 2005: 7) notes that, 'there is considerable evidence that social work does not have a good record in understanding or combatting family poverty'. This, it should be stressed, is only part of the picture; many social workers are acutely aware of the impact poverty and exclusion have on their clients and are passionately committed to alleviating them (Hooper *et al.*, 2007). Nonetheless, there is what Gill and Jack (2007) call 'poverty blindness'. One particularly sharp example of this is Brandon *et al.*'s (2009) finding that serious case reviews provided very little detail about the circumstances of families where children had died or suffered serious injury as a result of abuse, *'especially regarding whether they were living in poverty'* (p. 4, emphasis added). As is explored later in the book, child abuse and poverty are linked.

To try to understand why poverty blindness occurs, a good place to start might be where social workers begin to learn their trade. Perry (2005: 7) argues that there are 'far too few . . . social work education resources demonstrating the impact of poverty and social exclusion'. Similarly, Hooper *et al.* (2007: 116) conclude that organizations which train social workers:

> need to pay more attention to the many and complex ways in which poverty impacts on family life – appreciation of these is essential if practitioners are to engage families on low incomes in service provision and alleviate rather than increase social exclusion.

There is a gap here; hopefully this book will help to fill it.

Poverty is often thought of in monetary terms, as not having enough to provide a basic standard of living. However, research asking people living in poverty about their views suggests that, while money is crucial, there is more to it than this:

> When you haven't got a lot of money, you feel more deprived, excluded, isolated. You feel that you're in a rut and you can't get out because you've got no money. Having money would make a lot of people happy because you're always sort of struggling . . . it all sort of comes as a package.
>
> (Dawn, quoted in Strelitz and Lister, 2008: 14)

What do you think? 1.1: What is poverty?

To alleviate service users' poverty, social workers should be clear about what poverty is and how it damages lives. The quote by Dawn (above) suggests that, as well as not having enough money, poverty also involves feelings of isolation and exclusion. Three definitions of poverty are given in the table below. Read them and decide which you agree with and which you do not.

Table 1.1 Defining poverty

Would you say that someone in Britain is or is not poor if:		
1 They had enough money to buy the things they really needed but not enough to buy the things that most people take for granted?	Poor	Not poor
2 They had enough money to eat and live but not enough to buy other things they needed?	Poor	Not poor
3 They did not have enough money to eat and live without getting into debt?	Poor	Not poor

Source: adapted from Beresford et al. (1999: 50)

Comment

What you think poverty is will depend partly on your personal experience and values. For instance, many social work students have first-hand experience of poverty so are likely to have firm ideas about what it is. We discuss definitions more in Chapter 2 but for now two points to note about Dawn's definition are:

1 While she clearly thinks that lack of money is a big part of being poor there is also a social aspect involved, being 'isolated and excluded'.
2 Dawn also suggests that there is a psycho-social dimension: if people had more money so were not poor and excluded, that would make many of them happy.

As you read this book and think about poverty and social exclusion it might be useful for you to revisit these definitions and see if your views about what poverty is have changed.

Poverty and social exclusion are often used interchangeably and taken to mean much the same thing. The nature and definition of both concepts are discussed later but it is useful here to briefly discuss how the two concepts are related. While poverty is clearly associated with low income in wealthy societies, where few people starve, it is usually defined in relative terms; that is to say, 'poverty is less about shortage of income and more about the inability of people on low incomes to participate actively in society' (Ferragina *et al.*, 2013: 6). This is similar to social exclusion which Ferragina *et al.* (2013: 8) call a 'poverty-related term' which describes 'the process by which people, especially those on low incomes, can become socially, politically and economically detached from mainstream society'. As this suggests, social exclusion is sometimes presented as an effect of poverty and sometimes as a cause. The two concepts are similar and often overlap: 'some people experience material poverty and social exclusion simultaneously while others can be in poverty without being socially excluded or can be socially excluded without being poor' (Lister, 2004: 82–3).

For this book I conducted research with social workers in both children's and adult's services and in the voluntary and statutory sectors. Most of those who took part differentiated between poverty and social exclusion in ways similar to Lister's overlapping groups. One children's social worker said:

> I have to say with children with disabilities there is a level of social exclusion, sometimes it's accompanied by poverty but sometimes it's definitely not accompanied by poverty . . . [for example] some are excluded from their own families: grandparents, aunts, uncles, because they won't accept or appreciate that a child has got a disability, especially if the child has got something that is seen as socially challenging like autism.

On the other hand, many social workers spoke of children from impoverished families being socially excluded at school because they could not afford to take part in activities, ranging from breaks to school trips. At the other end of the age range, one social worker told me: 'Every older person I work with or have assessed is socially excluded. Very rarely is there someone who doesn't say to me, "I feel lonely, I've got no one around me." That's all the time, all the time.' In the academic literature social exclusion is seen as multi-dimensional, yet while it would not be safe to generalize too much from my research data, it does suggest that social workers see it in more straightforward terms and particularly as social isolation: lacking support from family and friends. There is probably a very practical reason for this; for all service user groups, having good, reliable social support networks is a key protective factor. Conversely, the more isolated people are the more vulnerable they are likely to be. This, of course, is why helping service users integrate into their communities is such an important part of social work practice.

Social exclusion was very prominent in social policy during the Labour government of 1997 to 2010. On taking office, the coalition government quickly dropped the term. However, while the term may have disappeared from use in Whitehall it all too plainly remains an 'empirical reality' outside the corridors of power: some 14 million people were estimated to be at risk of exclusion in 2011 (ONS, 2013a). Politicians' whims notwithstanding, such statistics do lend weight to Sheppard's (2006: 5) view that 'social exclusion is the very stuff of social work'.

Social exclusion is concerned with the social context of disadvantage: from what, how and why are people being excluded? Much the same is true of poverty: the forms it takes, the extent and causes of it, are shaped by the society in which it occurs. At a global level this is self-evident: poverty in Britain is very different from poverty in, say, Bangladesh. But it also applies at the local level of practice: understanding why service users are poor and excluded, what the likely consequences of that are and what can be done about it, requires awareness of the conditions in which they live. This is a theme of this book: exploring poverty and social exclusion in their context. In this introduction some general features of the current context are outlined, in part to show that while the need for anti-poverty practice is urgent, social workers are working in a cold climate: these are difficult times.

In the UK, early in the twenty-first century, poverty and social exclusion present new challenges to social work, for three reasons:

1 Both are getting much worse.
2 State welfare for deprived people is being withdrawn on an unprecedented scale.
3 Compared to what it has been in the past, the capacity of social work to respond to poverty and exclusion is restricted, especially in statutory services.

Evidence to support these points is set out in the following paragraphs (and at various points later in the book). I also go on to discuss how this unfavourable context relates to social workers' commitment to social justice.

For most of the twentieth century, Britain became a better place to live: living standards rose, health and life expectancy improved and we became a more equal society. That started to change in the 1980s when, with the election of a Conservative government in 1979, there began 'a thirty-year process of redistribution to the rich' (Levitas, 2012a: 320) and income inequality increased at an 'almost unprecedented rate' (Wilkinson, 1996: 94). This has brought historically high levels of poverty and inequality. The Labour government of 1997 to 2010 reduced child and pensioner poverty significantly and introduced many initiatives, not least Sure Start, to address social exclusion. Nonetheless, a review in 2010 found that 'Britain is an unequal country, more so than many other industrial countries and more so than a generation ago' (National Equality Panel, 2010: 1). Jordan and Drakeford (2012) argue that the economic crash of 2008 brought a radical change in social policy with former commitments to progressive redistribution (from rich to poor) and social inclusion being abandoned in favour of 'welfare discipline' and 'austerity'. This is evident in the coalition government's welfare reforms which include a cut of £20 billion from the benefits budget by 2015/16. These policies and the discourse of 'welfare dependency' which accompanies them have been characterized by Levitas (2012a: 322) as 'a neo-liberal shock doctrine providing an excuse for further appropriation of social resources by the rich'.

Formally the government is committed by legislation to eradicate child poverty by 2020. How seriously it takes this obligation is questionable given that: 'it seems impossible that the targets set out in the Child Poverty Act could be met, even if there were unprecedented changes in the labour market, welfare policy, and the amount of redistribution attempted by the state' (Browne *et al.*, 2013: 4). Worse, recent reductions in child poverty are likely to be reversed, with an estimated 3.1 million children living in poverty by 2020 (Browne *et al.*, 2013).

A review of the likely effects of welfare reform has found that 'poverty is expected to increase significantly more across the UK by 2015–16 than it would were the reforms not implemented' (UCL Institute of Health Equity, 2012: 10). Those most at risk include disabled people, single-parent families and some ethnic minority groups. In London it is estimated that between 82,000 and 133,000 households will be unable to afford their homes. Homelessness and overcrowding are likely to rise as is people moving within and between boroughs in search of affordable housing. The probable consequences of all this include:

- more suicides and attempted suicides; possibly more homicides and domestic violence
- an increase in mental health problems, including depression, and possibly lower levels of wellbeing
- worse infectious disease outcomes such as tuberculosis and HIV.
                                             (UCL Institute of Health Equity, 2012: 7)

London is not typical of the country generally – the cost of living is higher and groups vulnerable to poverty are over-represented in the capital. Nationally, however, it is estimated that in 2013 over half a million people were reliant on food aid (using food banks or receiving food parcels) and 4 million were in food poverty (Cooper and Dumpleton, 2013). Commenting on a surge in food bank use the chief executive of the Citizens Advice Bureau observed:

> Millions of families are facing a perfect storm of pressures on their budgets. The combined impact of welfare upheaval, cuts to public spending, low wages and the high cost of living are putting unbearable pressure on many households, forcing them to seek emergency help putting food on the table.
> (Gillian Guy, quoted in Citizens' Advice Bureau, 2013)

Austerity policies and cuts in funding for public services come at a time of rising need with the population increasing at both ends of the age range, young and old, the groups most reliant on social care. At its most extreme this leads to the situation depicted in the 'Barnet Graph of Doom', 'showing that within 20 years, unless things change dramatically, the north London council will be unable to provide any services except adult social care and children's services' (Brindle, 2012). This doomsday scenario is unlikely to be fully realized but the general contradiction between growing need for local authority social services and falling budgets has ominous implications. One is that as less essential but more popular services (libraries and leisure, for example) are cut, local people's support for care services will be eroded, widening further the social divide between disadvantaged people who rely on statutory services and better-off people who can afford private provision. Another implication is that this contradiction will give the spiral of tightening eligibility criteria a further twist: it will become harder to access services. Caught in this pincer, local authorities are likely to 'reconfigure' service delivery with more privatization, more charges and moving further from universal to targeted services. (Hannen, n.d.). A likely outcome of all this is that poor and excluded people will increasingly be left to rely on inadequate residual services.

These projections, about what might transpire, should not distract attention from what is already happening. Action for Children (2012) reports that its family support services are seeing more cases of suspected child neglect and an increase in the severity of the issues children face. Cuts in funding for children's services are falling hardest on preventive services and 'are most apparent in English urban areas and those authorities that have a high proportion of looked after children' (Chartered Institute of Public Finance and Accountancy, 2011: 5). Meanwhile, a 2012 survey of social workers found that:

> 85% have experienced notable cuts to services in the last 12 months and 78% have noticed jobs cuts or unfilled vacancies. Eligibility criteria has tightened, the use of unqualified staff is on the rise and caseloads are unmanageable for 77% of social workers.
>
> (BASW, 2012a: 6)

The government says it is determined to 'protect and support families of all shapes and sizes' (Secretary of State for Work and Pensions, 2012: 25). Yet one mother and service user sees the impact of austerity differently: 'Well, some of the families who are really struggling . . . they're going to be stuffed now, aren't they?' (anon., quoted in Action for Children, 2012: 10). Research by children's charities suggests this mother's view is more realistic. The charities found that while the introduction of Universal Credit will increase the income of some vulnerable families, this will not be enough to offset losses incurred by changes to other benefits and, perversely, the overall loss of income caused by welfare reform will be greatest for the most vulnerable families (Reed, 2012). Yet one social worker I interviewed, who works with vulnerable families, said: 'There are some families who, I honestly believe, if we gave them a hundred pound a week to lessen that anxiety: where they are low, they're depressed and everything, which impacts on the children . . . it would probably lift all that.' As it is, rather than getting extra money, the estimated combined impact of welfare reform and cuts in services is that vulnerable families will lose on average between £1,000 and £2,400 annually and the number of vulnerable families will rise (Reed, 2012).

Even in the extremely unlikely event that child poverty will be eradicated by 2020 the damage that poverty and social exclusion is doing now will have lasting effects, particularly in social inequalities in health. Health inequalities are differences, as measured by rates of illness and death, which occur between socio-economic groups. Put starkly, what this means is that poor people live shorter lives with more illness than rich people. For instance, while average male life expectancy nationally is 75 years, in one deprived part of Glasgow it is only 54, a 'health gap' of 21 years (Coren *et al.*, 2010).

Similar health inequalities confront social workers daily. Because they are poor and/or excluded, most service users are already ill or their health is threatened by their social situation. This has both practical and ethical implications: practical in that working to meet service users' basic material and social needs means addressing the social determinants of health; and ethical in that, 'to be true to its code of ethics, social work has a moral obligation to act when and where it can to oppose, reduce and mitigate the causes and consequences of health inequalities' (Bywaters, 2009: 364).

In much the same way as health inequalities, service users' poverty and social exclusion is both a practical and an ethical issue. It is practical in that poverty and social exclusion are usually underlying factors in the presenting issues which bring people into contact with social workers, they also restrict people's capacity to cope with such problems. As well as money, people who are poor also lack power and thus have less control over their lives and fewer options. This has a psychological impact, as explained by a service user:

> Talking about poverty is a very emotional thing for me. Money talks. Money is power. Because I don't have much money I always have to make choices, and there are limits on what I can give to my children. This makes me feel guilty.
>
> (Anon., quoted in Perry, 2005: 14)

The ethical dimension is that it is unjust that poor and excluded people are disempowered, stigmatized and suffer inequality in many areas of their lives. Social work is founded on a commitment to social justice. The BASW (2012b: 8) code of ethics states that: 'Social workers have a responsibility to promote social justice, in relation to society generally, and in relation to the people with whom they work.' Similarly The College of Social Work requires members to acknowledge that:

> . . . social work is founded on principles of social justice and I will therefore seek to understand and promote through my work outcomes that support human dignity and the respect of each member of society for their fellow human beings. I will challenge, in an appropriate manner, discrimination and stigmatisation wherever I encounter it.
>
> (The College of Social Work, 2013: 2)

While people become social workers for many reasons, it is often partly because the professional commitments to social justice accord with their personal ideals. However, social work is facing tough times. Even before austerity, Labour governments were in many ways 'tough on social work and tough on the values of social work' (Garrett, 2009: 1). The scope of statutory social work is increasingly restricted to reactive crisis intervention. In these circumstances social work agencies' policies and priorities can 'severely compromise a social worker's ability to act in accordance with her/his cherished beliefs' (Lymbery and Butler, 2004: 5). Making space for anti-poverty practice can then require a personal as well as a professional commitment. Lymbery and Butler rightly argue that social workers should resist organizational pressure to dilute their practice and that to do that they need 'strategies that will help them resist' (p. 5). A starting point for developing such strategies is to be critical, which involves 'taking an independent-minded approach to practice, and a willingness to take some risks' (Jordan, 2012: ix). Managerial imperatives, because they are often concerned with rationing scarce resources, tend to emphasize the control side of the 'care or control' tension in social work. Managerialism in social work, Lymbery (2004) notes, has two related aspects. First there is an acceptance that budgets are not adequate to meet needs for services and therefore budgetary constraints are introduced, accompanied by increased scrutiny of social workers' decision-making, to ensure compliance with tighter rationing. Second, and as a consequence, social work is increasingly bureaucratized and discretion is eroded. Hence the common complaint that social workers spend too much time in front of computers rather than in direct work with service users. This is not conducive to anti-poverty practice.

What do you think? 1.2: The experience of poverty and poverty awareness

In a project to develop poverty and social exclusion training for social workers (Perry, 2005), service users were asked what poverty meant to them. A selection of their answers is given in Table 1.2.

Table 1.2 'What does poverty mean to you?'

• (For some people) not being able to read and write and not having had a good education	• Lack of status
	• Feeling shame and stigma
	• Not having enough money or support
• Lack of power over your own life and a lack of choices	• Having a wealth of expertise in survival, courage and humility but this not being recognized
• Having no voice; not being heard	
• Having no right to refuse services that you feel are inappropriate	• Being blamed and judged by others for the situation you are in
• Having low self-esteem	

Source: Perry (2005: 18–19)

Questions for discussion

1 What do you think are the most significant aspects of the meaning of poverty identified by services users?
2 How do they relate to social work practice?

Comment

Perhaps the most significant point is the one about service users having a 'wealth of expertise in survival, courage and humility'. Recognizing that service users are 'experts by experience' can help build trust because you are acknowledging and building on their strengths. This can be the basis of working in partnership to address issues. In turn this can be empowering, helping service users change and gain some control over their situation.

Clearly because money, or the lack of it, is central to people's experience of poverty, income maximization is essential. Nowadays, social workers usually have a limited role in welfare rights work; it is usually done by specialists in other agencies. Nonetheless, social workers must be able to give good general advice. Moreover, income maximization and debt management will often involve very personal issues so should be approached sensitively, particularly given the stigma and low self-esteem that service users experience.

In the 'Right Trainers' project (Perry, 2005), service users identified many things they thought would help social workers to work constructively with people in poverty, including:

• being non-judgemental, caring, open-minded, genuine and not patronising;
• showing that you welcome families as human beings;
• acknowledging power differentials and having a commitment to minimizing them;
• understanding what is within parents' control and what is not.

Both Perry (2005) and Hooper *et al.* (2007) suggest that in social work education in anti-oppressive practice there is a need to pay more attention to the ways in which poverty and 'the accumulation of disadvantage over years, or even generations' (Hooper *et al.* 2007: 109) affects service users. Working under pressure, short of time and other resources, there can be a tendency for social workers to see poverty and social exclusion in pathological terms, resulting from service users' personal failings. This will not help service users cope with their situation and may well undermine any working relationship between social workers and their clients. The argument of this book is that poverty awareness, including an appreciation of the societal causes of poverty and exclusion, is essential to countering such damaging pressures.

Outline of the book

Broadly this book is divided into two main parts. Chapters 2 to 4 explore the context of social work with poor and excluded people. Chapter 2 looks at three aspects of poverty as it relates to social work: first, the causes of poverty; second, stigma and discrimination against poor people; and, third, agency: people's capacity to change their situation. Agency is relevant in two ways. First, it relates to the causes of poverty: do people behave in ways which brings poverty upon them? Second, how and to what extent can they take action to escape from poverty? In theoretical terms the issue is the interaction of agency, what people do, and structure – the wider social context which shapes and restricts poor people's options. Despite lacking power, status and money, service users can and do exercise agency to alleviate poverty; equally, social workers can and should exercise their agency to support service users doing that.

Social exclusion as a way of understanding multiple disadvantage is the focus of Chapter 3. Taking a historical perspective, the development of the concept is traced from the 'underclass debate' in the early 1990s to its centrality in the social policy of the Labour government of 1997 to 2010. The chapter explores what social exclusion is and how it can be tackled and applies the concept to three practice-related issues: whether there are 'neighbourhood effects' which worsen social exclusion in deprived areas; the significance of racism in causing the high rates of poverty of ethnic minority groups; and the social model of disability as a way of understanding and redressing the exclusion of people with disabilities.

Chapter 4 examines social changes associated with the idea that British society is broken. Perceived problems such as community breakdown and consumerism are related to neo-liberal globalization, as is the spread of managerialism, in the form of 'McDonaldization' in social work (Dustin 2007). All such 'social evils' are related to growing social inequality which is examined in two ways. First, inequalities in health are discussed as a social work issue because, as was discussed earlier, they particularly affect service users. Second, drawing on Wilkinson and Pickett's (2009) *The Spirit Level*, the chapter explores the relationship between high levels of inequality and social problems associated with poverty and social exclusion, which social workers often deal with, including teenage pregnancy.

The second part of the book, Chapters 5 to 7, looks at particular service user groups, respectively, children and families, older people and people in mental distress. There are two general themes here: how service users are affected by poverty and social exclusion and how social workers can address this. In Chapter 5 the relationship between poverty, exclusion and child abuse is explored. From this it is argued that practice with children and families should be informed by an ecological perspective to help social workers take account of the wider social factors which affect families. Social capital, the networks of social support families can draw on, is particularly important in resisting the effects of poverty and exclusion.

Chapter 6 discusses how older people are affected by social divisions and inequality. The interaction of the feminization of poverty and women's greater life expectancy renders women particularly vulnerable to social exclusion in old age. Simultaneously, with privatization there is a growing divide in social care services for older people, with poor people increasingly left to rely on tightly rationed residualized services.

In Chapter 7 it is argued that poverty and social exclusion both cause mental distress and are consequences of it. To show this the social construction of mental illness is analysed and applied to the entrenched inequalities experienced by Black people, in particular. Turning to responses to mental distress, the agency of the service user movement in developing recovery as an empowering process is discussed. This is then related to mutual aid and, thereby, to group work as a social work method which supports service users' and carers' collective self-help.

Chapter 8 discusses more general social work responses to poverty and social exclusion by developing three related themes. First, that social work's professional codes of ethics can be complemented by 'bottom up' values, specifically an 'ethic of care' and mutuality. Second, it is argued that in the practice context of high caseloads and rising thresholds for services, social workers need to 'make space' to be more able to ameliorate poverty and social exclusion. The third part of the argument is that to do this it is also necessary to move beyond the individualistic focus of most practice towards a more community-oriented approach. The Conclusion, Chapter 9, relates these themes to the current social and policy context by drawing parallels between the extreme poverty and exclusion that asylum seekers are forced to endure and similar, although less severe, hardship being imposed on poor people generally.

In part, this book is informed by primary research I conducted with nearly 40 social workers. The research was qualitative, semi-structured interviews and focus groups, exploring practice experiences of and responses to poverty and social exclusion. The sample included social workers in different teams and agencies, working with adults and with children and families, and in both the statutory and voluntary sectors. Although it is hoped that this sample gives a good picture of the variety of social workers' experiences, it is not representative. Hence the data has been used descriptively, for case studies and to illustrate particular points. As far as possible the case studies are presented in the social workers' own words in the hope that gives a better representation of their practice.

With austerity and welfare reform, poverty and social exclusion are growing in extent and severity. Seen from a health inequalities perspective, the effects of this will be to inflict illness and disability on service users and to shorten their lives. There could hardly be a greater imperative for social workers to be more 'poverty aware'. However, in the current context to use that understanding to inform practice is challenging. Social workers have to work in the contexts they find themselves and must observe the policies and practices the government and their employers require. Many social workers I interviewed were very poverty aware but frustrated by the constraints of managerialism. Yet often the direct work they described with service users seemed to endorse White's (2009: 143) point that 'opportunities for resistance can be found in the nooks and crannies within existing organisational frameworks'. Making space for anti-poverty practice will not change the world but it can make a significant difference to service users and carers.

2 Poverty and social work

Key messages

- Social workers should guard against 'povertyism', discriminating against people because they are poor, and be particularly wary of moralistic judgements about who is 'deserving' and 'undeserving' of support.
- How poverty is defined, measured and what its causes are believed to be are all linked and shape policy and practice responses to it.
- Living in poverty does influence people's attitudes and behaviour but there is little evidence to support the 'cycle of deprivation' and similar theories which hold that people cause their own poverty.
- The main causes of poverty lie in the unequal social and economic structures of society which reproduce and reflect social divisions of class, 'race', gender and disability, etc.
- Poor people, are not hapless victims, they can and do exercise agency, strive to cope with, and escape from poverty. This is particularly true of women.

> There can be no doubt that the poverty of the working classes of England is due, not to their circumstances . . . but to their improvident habits and thriftlessness. If they are ever to be more prosperous it must be through self-denial and forethought.
> (*Charity Organization Review*, 1881, quoted in Mooney, 1998: 64)

This quote from Victorian times is relevant here for two reasons. First, it has contemporary echoes in media and politicians' attacks on the 'dependency culture' of people who are alleged to prefer living on benefits rather than working for a living. Second, it is from the journal of the Charity Organization Society (COS), the organization from which British social work evolved. When these words were written it was not known how many people were poor but 20 years later surveys found that 'we are faced with the startling probability that from 25 to 30 per cent of the town populations of the United Kingdom are living in poverty' (Rowntree, 2000: 301). Then as now, poverty was widespread and poor people were being blamed for their own poverty by an organization which ostensibly was meant to help them.

The COS developed casework as a method of administering 'scientific philanthropy' to people who sought help from charities in Victorian Britain. At that time the only responsibility the state took for relieving poverty was through the 1834 New Poor Law by which relief was given on such harsh terms that its main function was to deter people from 'pauperism': the workhouse regime was so brutal that people would take even the worst, lowest paid work rather than seek Poor Law relief. Casework was complementary to this, used by charities to enforce a rigid distinction between the 'deserving' poor who they helped and the 'undeserving' who were left to the Poor Law. To do this casework involved a detailed investigation of a claimant's home life and general character (Mooney, 1998).

What do you think? 2.1: The 'deserving' and 'undeserving' poor

Table 2.1 provides summaries from COS records of cases that were investigated and either rejected as 'undeserving' or deemed 'deserving' and given help.

Questions for discussion

1 From the case summaries what general principles or criteria do you think were used to decide who was assisted and who was not?
2 There is an explicit moral agenda informing the COS decisions; do you think social workers today can, and should, be free of moral judgements when working with clients?

Table 2.1 'Deserving' and 'undeserving' cases

'Deserving' cases	'Undeserving' (rejected) cases
No. 3151. This was the case of a woman whose husband died suddenly, leaving her with a family of young children, one only a few days old. A grant in four weekly payments helped her until she was again able to undertake her usual occupation of a charwoman. No. 4056. This person, in consequence of long illness in her family, had been obliged to pledge her sewing machine [to a pawnbroker]; with some help from private sources (through the Society), she was enabled to redeem her machine and keep her work together. Case D. Widow, aged 67, with six children all grown up. Society granted temporary assistance; members of the Committee visited the case and induced the family to support their mother. Assistance now ceased.	Brighton COS alerted London COS about James Smith, an impostor who had lost his right hand and right leg, apparently in military service. They considered that other affiliated societies should be warned that Smith used his physical losses to win charitable hearts to supplement his 6d a day pension. A lamentable case of ingratitude and bad conduct illustrative of the difficulty of helping people whose vices prevent them helping themselves involved a man who had been financially assisted to buy a barrow which he had eventually sold for half its value and indulged in drink, judged by the COS to be his fatal propensity. A man stating that through slackness of trade, he had been out of work for months, applied for a loan of £2 to redeem from pawn clothing belonging to himself, his wife and three children, which he had parted with for food. He was found to be a widower, and the woman and the three children he mentioned did not belong to him. He was otherwise found to be undeserving.

Source: Mooney (1998)

Comment

There is a clear gender division here: women get helped, men usually do not. This reflects Victorian gender relations: it was seen as the male breadwinner's responsibility to provide for 'his' wife and family. If there was no man able to do this a woman might get assistance but even then it was likely to be short-term, intended to help the claimant help herself and no more. The moral agenda is also apparent in the last rejected case: because the man and woman were not married, the children 'did not belong to him' and the family were not helped. Generally, to be 'deserving', people had not only to be in need but also to be of good moral character, as judged by middle-class COS criteria.

Formally, social workers should put their personal prejudices aside when working with clients but being non-judgemental can be hard, especially amid constant media messages about 'scroungers' and 'skivers'. As Becker (1997: 116) argues, 'Social workers, like the public more generally, make distinctions and judgements between different groups of the poor, between the 'deserving' and 'undeserving' . . .'. For this reason social workers should be reflexive in the sense of being 'aware of the assumptions that underlie how they make sense of practice situations . . . [and] how relations of power are complicit in knowledge creation in social work practice' (D'Cruz et al., 2007: 77–8).

Stigma and povertyism

While social workers today are more aware of the social basis of poverty and exclusion than their nineteenth-century predecessors, they are still criticized for lacking poverty awareness (Gill and Jack, 2007). The legacy of Victorian philanthropy is apparent here both in methods and in attitudes and values. Casework, the predominant method in British social work, by its nature focuses on individuals and families so there is an inherent tendency not to recognize 'external' social and political factors. For a hard-pressed social worker it might, after all, appear easier and more logical to expect a poor family to change their behaviour rather than asking a welfare agency to change theirs. Yet, as Bob Holman (1978: 180) says, 'If the social worker's approach makes the poor feel more blameworthy, more inadequate, then they have allied themselves to the mechanisms which keep the poor at the bottom of a structured society.' This is 'povertyism', prejudice against poor people, which can take various forms including:

- having prejudiced, stereotypical, ideas about poor people, seeing them as feckless, irresponsible, or 'scroungers';
- blaming people for having problems caused by poverty e.g. being unable to cope on benefits while 'wasting money' on cigarettes.

Like other forms of discrimination, povertyism operates at individual, institutional and societal levels. Where social work agencies have long waiting lists and service users are made to wait for services they need urgently, it can reinforce the feeling that their views and needs are not taken account of by 'A system that can make them feel they don't matter' (Gupta and McNeill-Mckinnell, 2009: 63).

Povertyism in social work is a reflection of the stigma attached to poverty in society generally. Lister (2004: 101) relates this to 'othering', 'an on-going process . . . by which the line is drawn between 'us' and 'them' '. . . and through which a social distance is maintained'. That is, poor people are set apart by being presented and treated as different from, and inferior to, the non-poor. This has its roots in the 'deserving'/'undeserving' distinction of the Victorian Poor Law and philanthropy. A modern manifestation of this is the 'welfare dependency' discourse in which benefit claimants are depicted as idle and parasitic. A particularly noxious example was the portrayal of Mick Philpott, a long-term claimant who started a fire which killed six of his children, as a 'Vile Product of Welfare UK' (Dolan and Bentley, 2013). This newspaper headline was apparently endorsed by Prime Minister David Cameron's comments that the case raised 'wider questions about our welfare system . . . it shouldn't be there as a sort of lifestyle choice' (quoted in Groves, 2013). Given such messages, it might be expected that claimants are generally being seen as less deserving and therefore are more stigmatized (Bell, 2013). For poor people, however, the shame and humiliation of othering is 'painfully injurious to identity, self-respect and self-esteem' (Lister, 2004: 119).

What is poverty? Definitions and measures

Othering is a factor in 'the demoralisation, alienation and disintegration which may follow chronic stress arising from deprivation' (Baldwin and Spencer, 1993, quoted in Becker, 1997: 112). If it does such damage to service users good practice should obviously be based on a sound understanding of poverty. As Alcock (2006: 64) says, 'issues of definition, measurement, cause and solution are bound up together and an understanding of poverty requires an appreciation of the interrelationship between them all'. In other words, what we think poverty is (definition) will influence which people we recognize as being poor (measurement), why we think they are poor (causes), and what should be done about it (responses: policy and practice).

The first poverty surveys, of London by Charles Booth and of York by Seebohm Rowntree, used what are often called absolute or subsistence definitions: a person is poor if they do not have enough money to live on. Rowntree (2000: 87) argued that families were in 'primary poverty' if their income was insufficient 'to provide the minimum of food, clothing and shelter needful for the maintenance of merely physical health'. This was a deliberately harsh definition, intended to show that the experience of poverty was severe and so make a compelling case that something should be done about it. Consequently Rowntree (2000: 87) excluded what we would now see as essential to well-being: 'the mental, moral and social sides of human nature'.

Today, subsistence definitions are still used at a global level but in the UK relatively few people live on the cusp of starvation. In fact when Rowntree did his third survey of York in 1950, using a modified measure of his subsistence definition, he found that only 1.6 per cent of the population were in poverty. At the time this was taken as evidence that, with the creation of a universal welfare state after the Second World War, poverty had been 'abolished'. Poverty was however quickly 'rediscovered' in the 1960s. The person most responsible for this, Peter Townsend, went on to change how poverty in affluent societies was thought of. In his seminal work, *Poverty in the United Kingdom*, Townsend (1979: 31) redefined poverty in relative terms:

> Individuals, families and groups can be said to be in poverty when they lack the resources to obtain the types of diet, participate in the activities and have the living conditions and amenities which are customary, or are at least widely encouraged or approved, in the societies to which they belong.

The rediscovery of poverty and its redefinition as relative deprivation underlines the point that, because poverty is a social phenomenon its forms will change as society changes. With universal state welfare, full employment and rising living standards, British society in the 1960s was very different from Victorian times. Because Townsend's definition of poverty fitted so well with the changed social context it has been hugely influential. In the UK, government poverty statistics have been based on a relative definition ever since. And, as Bradshaw (2011a: 94) says, 'the international consensus that poverty is relative is really quite extraordinary'. Moreover, Townsend's definition of poverty foreshadowed social exclusion; people in relative poverty are, Townsend (1979: 31) argued, 'excluded from ordinary, living patterns, customs and activities'.

This is the essence of relative poverty: it is relative to the given social context and is based on income because without an adequate income people cannot participate in 'customary' social life. Much else flows from this, not least the understanding that 'social inequalities in health' are caused by lack of status and 'autonomy' is close to and based on a relative definition of poverty. Simply put, with money comes status and control over your life. In capitalist societies if you do not have money you will also want for respect and the power to decide your own fortunes. This will not be news to anyone who has lived on benefits for very long. You are effectively excluded from the mainstream and the psycho-social effects of this exclusion will take a toll on your health. Health inequalities and social work are discussed more in Chapter 4 – here the point is that because poverty is relative, shaped by its social context, the effects it has on service users are complex and profound: they go far beyond struggling to put food on the table.

An alternative way of defining poverty is Amartya Sen's capabilities approach. Sen questions the importance of income as the basis of poverty and argues that there is an absolute aspect to it. Central to Sen's analysis are 'functionings' and 'capabilities' where:

> A functioning is an achievement, whereas a capability is the ability to achieve. Functionings are, in a sense, more directly related to living conditions, since they are different aspects of living conditions. Capabilities, in contrast, are notions of freedom, in the positive sense: what real opportunities you have regarding the life you may lead.
>
> (Sen, 1987: 37)

For Sen it follows that poverty should be not be defined in terms of income but of 'the failure of basic capabilities to reach certain minimally acceptable levels' (Sen, 1992, quoted in Lister, 2004: 16). One value of this is that it allows a focus on individuals (rather than people on low incomes generally) and this can 'render gender inequalities more easily visible' (Lister, 2004: 17) because in families and households women's capabilities are often frustrated by men's power. Sen's approach is very influential in international development and is, Lister (2004) says, 'percolating through' in the global North. In Chapter 3, for example, reference is made to how Burchardt (2004) suggests it can be used in practice with disabled people. However, as Alcock (2006: 68) says, Sen's framework is 'rather abstract and philosophical' and probably because of that has never been satisfactorily operationalized (Bradshaw, 2011a).

To operationalize a definition of poverty is to apply it to the 'real world' of policy and practice, which usually starts with measuring how many people are poor. There are two linked and generally accepted ways of measuring relative poverty, both derived from Townsend's work. The first is through the use of a poverty index, a list of indicators made up of items intended to cover 'all the major areas of personal, household and social life' (Townsend, 1979: 251). The purpose is to measure the relationship between having the items and income. If the items in a poverty index give a broadly accurate representation of customary social life, it follows that people and households on lower incomes would have fewer of the items – which is what Townsend found. A related question is whether there is a poverty threshold: a level of income below which deprivation, lacking items in the poverty index and therefore lacking social participation, increases sharply. Townsend argued that there was such a threshold: at 150 per cent of the level of the main means tested benefit (then Supplementary Benefit). His argument was that this method of operationalizing his relative definition of poverty provided an objective poverty threshold: a line against which the number of people in poverty could be counted based on how people on low incomes actually lived.

What do you think? 2.2: Relative poverty and necessities

One criticism of Townsend's method was that in compiling the poverty index no allowance was made for why people did not have items: was it by choice or because they could not afford them (Gordon and Pantazis, 1997). In response to this criticism a second, *consensual*, method of measuring relative poverty was developed. This uses data from social surveys which ask three key questions:

1 What items do people think are necessities?
2 Whether they had those necessities?
3 If they did not was that because they did not want them or could not afford them?

From this a poverty index is compiled which is consensual in that the items included are seen as necessities by a majority (50 per cent or more) of the population. There have been four surveys using this method: in 1983, 1990, 1999 and 2012, so we can see how attitudes about what people should have in order not to be poor have changed. In Table 2.2 are a selection of the indicators used in the surveys; it includes some items which most people think are necessities and some which they do not.

Table 2.2 Poverty index: necessities of modern life?

Item	Necessity: yes or no?
Two meals a day (for adults)	
Telephone (landline)	
Car	
Home computer	
Mobile phone	
Internet access	
Two pairs of all-weather shoes	
Roast joint or equivalent once a week	
Holiday away from home	
New, not second-hand, clothes (adults)	
Presents for family or friends once a year (Christmas or birthdays)	

Source: adapted from PSE (2013)

Questions for discussion

1 In your opinion which items in the table are necessities: things people should have so as not to be in relative poverty?
2 Given how 'customary social life' has changed in recent times how do you think public attitudes might have changed about which items are necessities and which are not?

Comment

What we might think is necessary for normal social participation is influenced by many things, not least by how people in our own social circle live and by media messages. The items in Table 2.2 were selected because they illustrate two broad changes (see Table 2.3 for the details):

1 Rising living standards and especially changes in technology. Support for mobile phones, home computers and internet access as necessities has increased greatly since the 1990s, although they are still not seen as necessities by most people.
2 That in 2012, with the economic downturn and austerity, there was a lowering of expectations about some items which previously had growing support. In particular two items which a majority had seen as necessities now have only minority support:

a) presents for family or friends once a year (Christmas or birthdays);
b) a holiday away from home (once a year).

These contradictory trends have implications for understanding how poor and excluded people live. One issue with this consensual method is how accurately public opinion reflects how people actually live: is there a difference between what people think are necessities and customary behaviour? According to the survey, mobile phones are not necessities yet in 2013 92 per cent of adults in the UK had a mobile phone and 51 per cent had a smartphone. Also, people in lower socio-economic groups are more likely to live in 'mobile-only' homes, partly because of the cost implications (Ofcom, 2013). So, contrary to the survey results, the evidence is that mobile phones are very much a part of customary social life, especially for poor people. In the research for this book a family centre social worker described the significance young mothers attached to mobile phones:

> On the whole people struggle to manage – but always manage to have a phone . . . It's a priority for young people to have an up-to-the-minute mobile phone, even when they've not got much money coming in . . . I think people would eat less to have a phone . . . it's really, really important to be in touch with people all the time. I can understand, if you're very young and got a baby and stuck in some horrible flat, you can communicate with people outside: it takes you out of yourself, it's an escapism. It's important for them . . . They come and show us, 'Oh look I've got this one, it's £100'!

Table 2.3 Poverty index: changes in necessities

Item	Previous surveys	2012
Two meals a day (adults)	64% (1983)	91%
Telephone (land line)	43% (1983)	77%
Car	22% (1983)	44%
Home computer	5% (1990)	40%
Mobile phone	8% (1999)	40%
Internet access	6% (1999)	41%
Two pairs of all-weather shoes	78% (1983)	54%
Roast joint or equivalent once a week	67% (1983)	36%
Holiday away from home	63% (1983)	42%
New, not secondhand, clothes (adults)	64% (1983)	46%
Presents for family or friends once a year (Christmas or birthdays)	63% (1983)	46%

Source: adapted from PSE (2013)

Another way of measuring poverty is by income-based poverty lines: people whose income is below a given amount are deemed to be poor. There are several such poverty lines but the most widely used is the 'Households Below Average Income' (HBAI) measure. This is usually set at 60 per cent of the average (median) household income. To slightly complicate things there are two versions of the HBAI standard: before and after housing costs. Anti-poverty campaigners tend to prefer the after housing costs measure because it gives a better picture of how much income people actually have to spend (see Aldridge et al., 2012). In calculating how many people are below this poverty threshold, incomes are adjusted to take account of household composition. Table 2.4 shows how much money, on the 60 per cent threshold, different household types have to spend each week.

The HBAI poverty line is arbitrary in that it is not directly based on any calculation of how much money households need to avoid being in relative poverty. This has however been done with the Minimum Income Standard: 'the minimum acceptable standard of living in Britain today that includes, but is more than just, food, clothes and shelter. It is about having what you need in order to have the opportunities and choices necessary to

Table 2.4 Household incomes at 60 per cent HBAI poverty line 2010/11

Family composition	Low-income threshold before housing costs (BHC) £ per week	Low-income threshold after housing costs (AHC) £ per week
Single with no children	168	125
Couple with no children	251	215
Lone parent with two children under 14	269	211
Couple with two children under 14	351	301

Source: Aldridge et al. (2012: 15)

participate in society' (Aldridge *et al.*, 2012: 19). For a 'working age family' the HBAI poverty line is about 28 per cent lower than the Minimum Income Standard. In other words the HBAI threshold is a bit like Rowntree's primary poverty: people who are poor by this measure are very poor indeed, a point to bear in mind when looking at the figures below.

The Labour government of 1997 to 2010 made reducing child poverty a priority and gave it legislative force in the Child Poverty Act 2010, which commits the government to 'eradicate' child poverty by 2020. Obviously, to assess progress towards this goal we need to know how many children are poor at different times. The statistics show that Labour did reduce child poverty significantly:

- by the 60 per cent HBAI *before* housing costs measure, 1.1 million children were lifted out of poverty between 1996/97 and 2010/11;
- by the *after* housing costs measure progress was slower, child poverty falling by 700,000 over the same period.

(Stewart, 2012)

As is discussed in Chapter 4, poverty is both a determinant of child wellbeing and a causal factor in child abuse. Since most child abuse passes under the radar of children's services, reducing poverty is a vital preventive measure. Labour's success in reducing child poverty, while not above criticism, does show how definitions, measures and policy and practice are linked: the likelihood is that the wellbeing of many children will have been improved and their risk of being abused reduced because they have been lifted out of poverty.

What do you think? 2.3: Reducing poverty: 'deserving' and 'undeserving' social groups?

While child poverty gets most attention the wellbeing of people of all ages is damaged by poverty. Figure 2.1 shows recent trends in poverty by age groups, with marked reductions for children and pensioners but a sizeable increase for childless working-age adults. These trends are partly a reflection of the political priority given to different groups.

Questions for discussion

1 Do you think politicians (and the electorate) think some age groups are more 'deserving' than others, and if so, why is that?
2 If that is the case what might it imply for social work with working-age adults in particular?

Comment

The think-tank Demos (n.d.) points out that while children and pensioners 'are exempt from the evermore prevalent narrative of the deserving and undeserving poor', working-age adults are not. As a consequence they are largely ignored in policy and have become the fastest growing group in poverty. They are also

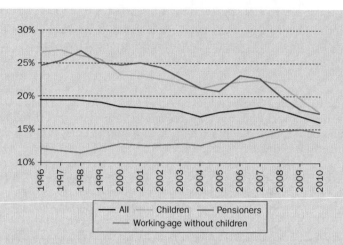

Figure 2.1 Relative poverty by age group (%) 1996 to 2010
Source: Joyce and Sibieta (2013)

particularly vulnerable, 'most likely to be transformed by life events' (Demos, n.d.). Research shows that working-age adults are a diverse group but include what Wood *et al.* (2012) call 'insecure singles': people living on their own, usually in rented housing and who are often unemployed and on low incomes. They are also 'highly likely to experience physical and mental health problems . . . [and] live in the most deprived neighbourhoods and receive mixed levels of support from neighbours and family' (Wood *et al.* 2012: 49). Because of this social exclusion 'insecure singles' are likely to fall foul of the government policy agenda which reinforces distinctions between the 'deserving' and 'undeserving' poor, largely based on 'a work–non-work axis', in which people who are not working are presented as 'dependent, irresponsible and arguably even . . . second-class citizens' (Patrick, 2012: 9). In terms of meeting need, the consequences of this othering are severe:

> . . . the historic underfunding of care is being exacerbated by cuts to local authority funding and leading councils to remove care and support from all but a minority of those with the seemingly most complex needs . . . Four in ten are failing to have their basic needs met, and underfunding is turning back the clock on disabled people's independence: nearly half of disabled adults report services aren't supporting them to get out into the community.
>
> (Brawn *et al.*, 2013: 6)

One purpose of measuring poverty is to shed light on its causes: why people are poor. This is a thorny, inherently political, question to which there are many different approaches. Alcock (2006) usefully condenses these into two general perspectives: *pathological* where the characteristics of poor people are said to cause their poverty and *structural* views which see the primary causes of poverty as lying in wider socio-economic and political forces.

Causes of poverty: pathological theories

Perhaps the two most influential pathological theories are Oscar Lewis' 'culture of poverty' theory and the 'cycle of deprivation' thesis expounded by Keith Joseph when he was (Conservative) Secretary of State for Social Services in 1972. The essence of both is the claim that poor people, families and communities, have or develop a different culture from mainstream society and it is this that causes and perpetuates their poverty, because it shapes their behaviour and attitudes, as summarized by Holman (1978: 107):

> Unmotivated and helpless people do not work their way out of poverty. Those unwilling to postpone pleasures do not save. Change will never come if they are unwilling to organise . . . inevitable poverty does not breed resentment because the culture of poverty is a way of accepting poverty.

The cycle of deprivation thesis emphasizes the role of the family, and child development, in transmitting such attitudes and behaviour across generations. While Keith Joseph recognized socio-economic factors, his concern was with the 'casualties of society': 'the problem families, the vagrants, the alcoholics, the drug addicts, the disturbed, the delinquent and the criminal' (Joseph, 1972, quoted in Coffield *et al.*, 1980: 2). They were, he claimed, 'inadequate people who tend to be inadequate parents and inadequate parents tend to rear inadequate children' (Joseph, 1972, quoted in Coffield *et al.*, 1980: 1). Among the consequences of this were that the children would probably fail in school, have unstable relationships and marriages and, lacking ambition and motivation, end up unemployed or in low-paid jobs. They would thus grow up and live in poverty much the same as their parents had, and likely pass that inheritance on to their own children (see Figure 2.2).

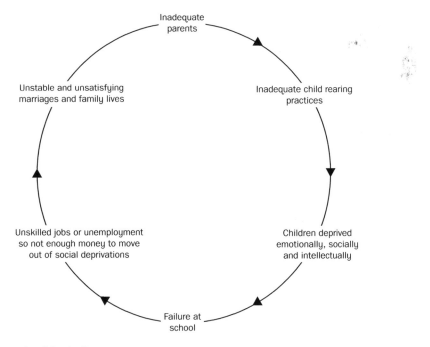

Figure 2.2 The cycle of deprivation

Source: Holman (1978: 117)

There are three main criticisms of cultural theories of poverty. The first is that research shows that poverty is generally not transmitted across generations. Research into the 'cycle of deprivation' theory found that 'most of the children from poor homes did not repeat the poverty of their families and communities, and that most of those who became poor did not themselves come from such deprived backgrounds' (Alcock, 2006: 39). Second, there is also little evidence that a distinct culture of poverty exists to the extent that advocates of the theory suggest. This lack of evidence notwithstanding, cultural explanations regularly resurface. One manifestation of this, the 1990s 'underclass debate', is examined in Chapter 3. Currently a key aim of the coalition government's welfare reform agenda is to end a supposed 'culture of dependency':

> . . . where you could easily be better off on benefits than trying to find work . . . In order to give people back their hope, aspiration and self respect we are sending a clear message: it is no longer OK to opt out of a life of work . . . We are ending the something for nothing culture.
>
> (Osborne and Duncan Smith, 2012)

In fact, recent research into the lives of people living on the margins of poverty in Middlesbrough, for instance, found that, 'despite repeated returns to unemployment and repeated engagement in only poor work participants retained a strong commitment to employment' (Shildrick *et al.*, 2012: 5).

The third criticism of cultural explanations is not so much about the extent of poverty but more about its causes. Bob Holman, a former social worker, rejects cultural explanations of poverty but recognizes:

> that *some* of the poor do display attitudes and behaviour which appear to reinforce their condition, that *some* cycles of deprivation can be identified and that the child rearing methods of *some* poor parents do not seem in the best interests of their children.
>
> (Holman, 1978: 137, emphasis in original)

Among the children's social workers interviewed for this book, there was near unanimity that there is a cycle of deprivation by which poverty is reproduced among some families. One child protection social worker, for example, recounted the reply of a 13-year-old boy when she asked him why he did not stop smoking and taking drugs: 'He said to me, he was conceived in cigarettes and drugs, he was born in it, he was raised in it and he was still living in it . . . so why would he change?'

Holman (1978) suggests three reasons why this happens:

1 That rather than resulting from long past inadequate parenting, parents may 'fail' because of recent prolonged adversity, in, for instance, education, housing or employment.
2 That poor parenting might be a response to deprivation rather than what the parents might wish for their children: 'Faced with material anxieties, accommodation difficulties and other distressing problems some parents could not cope properly with their children' (Holman, 1978: 138).
3 That services play a part in 'exaggerating or formulating the apparent deficiencies of the poor' (Holman, 1978: 139). In education, for instance, Bernard Coard described how West Indian working-class children are 'made educationally sub-normal' by the white, middle-class culture of schools which can leave a child 'feeling that he is somehow inferior, and bound to fail' (Coard, 1971, quoted in Richardson, 2007: 37).

Holman's argument is that 'cultures of poverty' are produced not by the moral or behavioural failings of poor people but by the powerful social forces which shape and limit their lives.

Causes of poverty: structural theories

This brings us to structural perspectives on poverty. The starting point of structural theories is that society is organized (or structured) unequally; the distribution of power, status, wealth and income is stratified: people at the top have more and people at the bottom less. Two things follow from this: first, poverty is relational in the sense that it cannot be understood in isolation from the totality of social relations, rich, poor and all those in between. Second, that social institutions function to maintain and reproduce this structured inequality.

Structural theories of poverty, often influenced by Marxism, are primarily concerned with the economic basis of social relations. Jones and Novak (1999: 18–19) argue that poverty in its current form is a product of capitalism. That is not to say that there was no poverty or inequality in earlier times but that the class relations specific to capitalism give contemporary poverty its particular character:

> The private ownership of wealth that characterises capitalist production, the ownership of the land, factories, machinery, offices and shops on which the majority depend for their employment thus frames the condition of poverty, and together these two seemingly natural, but in reality historically specific, features provide the dynamic through which capitalism has developed.

From a structural perspective, poverty is also functional for capitalism in two ways. First, the poor act as a 'reserve army of labour' to be sucked into and expelled from employment as changing economic conditions require. Second, it has a disciplinary effect: in British society this was most explicit in the 1834 New Poor Law where the brutal workhouse regime was designed to instil the discipline of wage labour into the newly-emerging industrial working class (Novak, 1988). Adherence to discipline depends, of course, on attitudes and values and in that sense is a moral question. Hence early social workers, using the COS casework method to separate the 'deserving' from the 'undeserving' poor, were functional to nineteenth-century industrial capitalism, their compassion notwithstanding.

In the decades after the Second World War the functional nature of poverty was ameliorated by state welfare and full employment. This changed from the 1980s with de-industrialization, globalization and the transition to a 'flexible labour market' (see Chapters 4 and 6). With these changes we moved into a new period of persistently high rates of poverty, as shown in Figure 2.3. The graph also shows that while poverty has remained high, over 12 million people annually, the proportion on very low incomes, (less than 40 per cent HBAI) has steadily increased, now comprising two fifths of those in poverty.

An unusual feature of this growth of poverty is that employment has increased: more people are working but this is not necessarily freeing them from poverty. Whereas in the mid-1980s less than a third of children in poverty were in working families, by 2012 60 per cent of poor children lived in families where at least one adult was working (Aldridge, 2012). Both Labour and the coalition governments have promoted work as the best 'route out of poverty' but, as Shildrick *et al.* (2012) found for those trapped in the 'low-pay, no-pay cycle', 'poor work did not provide stepping stones to better employment and

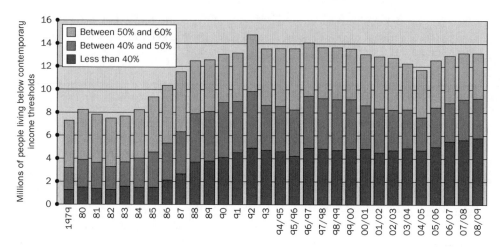

Figure 2.3 UK Poverty: 1979 to 2008/9
Source: Parekh et al. (2010: 27)

security in adulthood' (p. 5) . While the nature of post-industrial Middlesbrough's labour market was the main causal factor of this, ill health and caring responsibilities also limited people's employment options. This, however, is a manifestation of social inequalities in health as the nature of the jobs available 'could also generate ill health which served to then limit people's availability for jobs: poor work made people ill' (Shildrick *et al.*, 2012: 143).

Despite growing evidence that 'low paid, menial and insecure work does not deliver the much hyped rewards and, conversely, insecure work for poverty wages can actually harm family life and individual wellbeing' (Patrick, 2012: 7) the disciplinary function of poverty is increasingly evident in social policy discourses and practice. In the distress and harm inflicted on disabled people by the Work Capability Assessment there are clear echoes of the New Poor Law (Bambra, 2008). This is legitimized by a discourse which seeks to stigmatize those not working as undeserving 'scroungers'. Integral to this are pathological explanations of poverty as in the coalition's welfare reform strategy which claims that 'the root causes of poverty . . . [are] family breakdown; educational failure; drug and alcohol addiction; severe personal indebtedness; and economic dependency' (Duncan Smith, 2010: 1). Such 'root causes' might more usefully be seen as problems caused or compounded by poverty and social exclusion. Equally, structural factors such as low pay, zero hour contracts, underemployment and austerity are noticeably absent from Duncan Smith's list.

Structural theories of poverty are usually concerned with class; however if poverty is structural in that, to quote Holman (1978: 239) its 'main function is regarded as upholding prevailing social and economic structures' they can also be applied to other social divisions including, for example, 'race' and gender.

The much higher rates of poverty that most black and minority ethnic (BME) groups suffer is discussed more in Chapter 3. However, Law (2012: 198) notes that recent research has found that the causes of this include 'persistent discrimination, patterns of educational qualification, labour-market outcomes [and] housing locations'. These are structural factors which result, for instance, in nearly half of all young Black people being unemployed compared to only a fifth of white men. As the National Equality Panel

(2010: 234) found: 'the central problem in relation to racial equality and the labour market is now unequal levels of unemployment, and the employment sectors which some people are constrained to enter . . . [with] clear evidence of discrimination in recruitment'.

In relation to the 'feminization of poverty', Millar (2009: 121–2) explains that:

> Poverty is more likely to be found among people who do not have jobs and where no-one in the household has a job, who have long-term health problems or disabilities, who have large families, who are sole-parent families, who come from ethnic minority groups . . . and who are elderly or live alone. In each case, it is women who have higher rates of poverty than men, and this has been true for many years.

Here too the structural dimensions are complex, working in different ways in different spheres. Within the home, for example, patriarchy in the form of the unequal control and distribution of household income can cause women to be economically dependent, because they do more unpaid caring than men, which can result in women's poverty being hidden within household income (Lister, 2004). Outside the home the feminization of poverty 'is strongly influenced by the prevalence of precarious work, with low wages and insecure employment particularly affecting women's poverty rates' (Garthwaite, 2010).

Agency and structure

One question that arises from structural explanations is: where does people's behaviour fit in? Holman (1978: 239) makes the important point that structural poverty 'compels behaviour and provokes adaptions which reinforce the social deprivations of the poor'; 'cultures of poverty' are an example of this. However, a danger of emphasizing structural influences on behaviour is that it can imply that poor people are hapless victims of circumstance who have little choice but to accept their fate. This, of course, is wrong; rather the issue is the relationship between structure and agency: 'the capacity of people to be creative, reflexive human beings . . . to be active agents in shaping their lives, experiencing, acting upon and reconstituting the outcomes . . . in relation to wider forms of stratification and social relations of power' (Williams *et al.*, 1999, quoted in Lister, 2004: 127).

People can act individually and collectively to change their situation and, in doing so, can change structures. The development of the service user movement and its influence on changing how services are delivered and on what terms is testament to this. Lister (2004) identifies four types of agency exercised by people in poverty:

1 getting by;
2 getting (back) at;
3 getting out;
4 getting organized.

'Getting by' is day-to-day coping, the 'fight to keep going' which is often not recognized as a form of agency. The 'Hunger Hurts' blog illustrates this powerfully:

> Tomorrow, my small boy will be introduced to the world of pawnbroking, watching as his mother hands over the TV and the guitar for an insulting price, but something towards bridging the gap between the fear of homelessness, and hanging in for a week or two more. Trying to consolidate arrears, red-topped

letters, and bailiffs, with home security, is a day to day grind, stripping back further the things that I can call my own.

(Monroe, 2012)

This perhaps is the type of agency that most immediately confronts social workers because, as Lister (2004) says, 'the cloak of invisibility' is often only lifted when it breaks down: when an individual or family can no longer cope and hit a crisis. 'Getting by' is associated with 'resilience and resourcefulness' which can be both personal and social. It is also usually associated with managing money, where there are two main strategies: 'ball-juggling and debt' or 'tight money control and cutting back'. These are not mutually exclusive, of course, and can be very demanding, requiring skill and effort to do things which in better-off families happen as a matter of course – keeping food on the table, for instance. Getting by is not just about money. Poverty does not spare you the 'biographical problems', illness, accidents, relationship problems, etc., that everyone encounters, it just makes them harder to cope with. In doing this social resources, particularly support networks, can be crucial. This is both gendered, mainly done by women, and reciprocal: whether emotional, practical or material, 'drawing on social resources is an active process of giving as well as receiving' (Lister, 2004: 137).

Resistance is the essence of Lister's 'Getting (back) at' type of agency. The 2011 riots which mainly involved socially excluded young people are an example of this. As Lister (2004: 140) notes, 'the anger and despair felt by some who feel trapped in poverty can explode into destructive forms of agency'. More common 'everyday resistance' might involve unemployed claimants doing unreported work, generally resisting or subverting the conditions attached to social security benefits and rejecting or challenging the stigma of poverty.

The two main ways of 'getting out' of poverty are via education and employment. However, as we have seen, finding work is becoming an increasingly associated with the 'low-pay, no-pay cycle' often bringing only temporary respite from poverty. The case study in Chapter 4 (What do you think? 4.4) shows one mother's determination to escape poverty by improving her education and by working shifts. That this is not easy is evident in the stress it created for the family. It also illustrates other aspects of agency: how people use different forms of agency simultaneously (collective coping strategies with childcare to support the mother's attempts to 'get out') and how it is gendered.

The last of Lister's forms of agency is 'getting organized'; this probably most often takes the form of collective self-help which can grow out of informal support networks. It is a form of community action which Lister (2004: 154) says typically addresses 'the needs of children and young people, lack of local amenities, environmental problems and debt'. Although there is not space to discuss it here, the Disabled People's Movement is also, in many ways, a manifestation of getting organized to challenge poverty (see e.g. Beresford, 1996).

What do you think? 2.4: 'Getting organized': credit unions and agency

In the extract below Ledwith (1997: 49–50) describes the development of a credit union in a deprived and stigmatized community:

> Unsurprisingly, it was the women of the credit union who rolled their sleeves up and transformed the idea into a reality . . . They developed skills they never dreamt they had. They identified other women from the

community and, in this way, the band of volunteers grew. They staffed collection points, pored over the bookkeeping, and assessed people for loans . . .

A credit union is founded on cooperation, mutuality and trust, encouraging its members to participate in policy making and to take an active interest in the day-to-day procedures . . . It serves the financial needs of the community by encouraging regular saving to provide a common pool for loans, and education is part of its role. This is the principle of mutuality upon which the system works – savings must remain intact when a loan is taken out, otherwise the pool is depleted.

. . . As confidence grew the credit union women played a key role in travelling far and wide to other community groups to support them in establishing their own credit unions . . . This process was immensely empowering. Communities in poverty usually believe that they are alone in their suffering, and the collective action generated by this anti-poverty movement brought confidence and optimism.

Questions for discussion

1 Ledwith (1997) emphasizes the agency of women in the success of the credit union. If women are more likely than men to take the lead in mutual aid activities, why do you think that is?
2 Can you suggest some reasons why social workers should support credit unions?

Comment

Ledwith's argument about women and mutual aid is based on gendered patterns of caring and the 'feminization of poverty': because it is usually their immediate responsibility women are first to react to threats, such as loan sharks, to 'home, family and community'.

Drakeford and Gregory (2008: 146) argue that promoting credit unions 'ought to be a part of any social worker's effort to assist in that everyday struggle which users face in managing the chronic conditions of persistent poverty'. Credit unions are better able to do this if they expand their activities beyond the traditional loans secured against savings to offer instant loans and help with budgeting and debt management. Also encouraging service users to get involved in credit unions can help overcome social isolation.

Poverty dynamics

The interaction of agency and structure is apparent in 'poverty dynamics': people's movements in and out of poverty, which are determined both by individuals' actions and by prevailing social and economic conditions. Most poverty statistics give a 'snapshot' picture of how many people are poor at one point in time, and this can give the false impression that the poor and 'non-poor' are two fixed and separate groups. In fact there is constant movement between the two groups so snapshot figures underestimate how many people are affected by poverty. For example, while the average rate of poverty between 1991 and 1998 was 15 per cent of the population, during that period twice as many people (31 per cent) were poor at least once (Smith and Middleton, 2007). Poverty dynamics are useful in understanding why individuals and families become poor partly because they shed light on the importance of household resources in people's vulnerability to poverty; this in turn gives pointers to factors which can help people escape from poverty.

There are two general aspects to what causes particular households to fall into poverty (Smith and Middleton, 2007: 5):

> the social characteristics or personal resources of an individual or household which mediate how resistant or vulnerable they are to poverty, and the event which actually triggers entry into poverty. What triggers poverty for some will not trigger it for others.

Among social characteristics, educational attainment is a protective factor whereas previous experience of poverty is a risk factor: people who have been poor once are more likely to be poor again. Triggers are the events which alter the balance between household needs and the income needed to meet them, and there are two types:

1 Changes in household income – the main factors here are work related: mainly losing or getting a job, followed by wage cuts or rises.
2 Changes in household size, typically either by having more children or by a two-parent family becoming a one-parent family.

Triggers for men are more likely to be income related whereas for women household size is more significant (Smith and Middleton, 2007). Although women are more vulnerable than men, 'not being white' carries a three times greater risk of being poor than does being a woman (Tomlinson and Walker, 2009). Many people, of course, are never poor and most people who become poor escape relatively quickly. But a minority, less than 1 in 10 people according to Jenkins (2011) suffer persistent long-term poverty. And the longer people are poor the less likely they are to escape it (Smith and Middleton, 2007).

'Escape', though, is probably the wrong word. There is a 'rubber band' model of poverty dynamics: most people's incomes fluctuate but rarely move far from a long-term average, and if they do, after a while the rubber band will probably snap them back to that average (Ridge and Millar, 2011). This is linked to 'churning', or recurrent poverty, as in the 'low-pay, no-pay cycle'. For people trapped in this dynamic, getting a job may raise their income enough to lift them just over the poverty line but the job will probably not last and, crucially, the time spent above the poverty line will often not be 'enough for people to build up their material resources to the point where they have a meaningful impact on their well-being and security' (Smith and Middleton, 2007: 3). They will thus be vulnerable to further triggers which might plunge them back into poverty.

In understanding how these dynamics affect service users, a life course perspective, taking account of the cumulative impact of life events and how they can render people vulnerable at key transition points (see Chapter 4) can highlight:

> . . . that employment history constitutes both periods of employment and transitions between employment. For many, these transitions will be interspersed by periods out of employment, for example unemployment, to undertake childcare or illness. Currently, these points of transition represent 'flash points' for entering poverty. For example, loss of work is the most common trigger of poverty,

movement from a two- to lone-parent household often coincides with job loss, and children with a parent moving in and out of illness are just as disadvantaged as those with persistently ill parents.

(Smith and Middleton, 2007: 90)

As this quote suggests, poverty dynamics are linked to social inequalities in health, and the onset of disability or ill health, for instance, is often a trigger. But the causal relationship between poverty and ill health works in both directions: 'people who become disabled are more likely to have been in poverty before the onset of an impairment than those who do not become disabled' (Smith and Middleton, 2007: 6). Seen from a life-course perspective the process can be cumulative: poverty and illness or impairment compounding each other over time.

Coming back to the interaction of structure and agency, Tomlinson and Walker (2010: 5) conclude that, 'while personal attributes and circumstances contribute significantly to determining the risk of recurrent poverty, they are overshadowed by structural factors that shape the opportunities for financial security offered by the labour market'. Debate about poverty and its causes is inherently political because it questions the distribution of power and resources in society. At the time of writing, the coalition government is conducting a consultation on how to change the measurement of child poverty. It wants to replace the current income based (HBAI) poverty measures with a 'multi-dimensional indicator', a single number which will give 'a better representation of the reality of children's lives' (Duncan Smith, 2012). The dimensions suggested include income but also factors like parental skill level, family stability and parental health. As many social workers know, the latter are associated with poverty, but they are not *measures*. Living on a low income does undermine the functioning of a minority of families, but not of the majority. A likely outcome of these 'inept and confused' proposals (Bradshaw and PSE Team 2013: 2) is that the new 'measure' will give a much lower rate of poverty because it includes 'worklessness', so the two thirds of poor households where at least one person is in work could be excluded. This would make it easier for politicians to claim they are meeting their obligation to 'eradicate' child poverty, even as it increases (Garnham, 2013).

It is probably not a coincidence that the government want to move away from income-based poverty lines when it is in the process of cutting £20 billion from benefits; cuts which will severely test the coping strategies of many service users. A key reason for using income-based poverty measures is that income underpins wellbeing. If children and adults are pushed deeper into poverty their ability to participate in society will suffer, as will their physical and mental health. In asserting that the main causes of poverty are pathological and looking to change how poverty is measured while cutting benefits, the government is demonstrating the truth of Alcock's (2006: 64) point, mentioned earlier, that 'issues of definition, measurement, cause and solution are bound up together'.

Solutions, in the form of anti-poverty practice, can be challenging, particularly in the current climate. However, social workers, like service users, can also exercise agency. This is particularly pertinent to statutory services which are often bureaucratic. Bureaucracy and lack of resources are major impediments to anti-poverty practice. It can be difficult, as Wilks (2012: 77) says, 'to act ethically in circumstances where the scope for independent autonomous decision making is limited'. Yet space can be made to act on ethical commitments to social justice and empowerment as, for instance, in what White (2009) calls 'quiet challenges'. A community orientation, which involves building alliances with service users and other professionals, can assist in this. These points are explored more in Chapter 8. Here the point is that even in difficult circumstances social workers can, should and do exercise agency to tackle poverty and social exclusion.

Summary of main points

- Social work originated in attempts to impose moralistic distinctions between the 'deserving' and 'undeserving' poor. Similar discriminatory processes, 'povertyism' and 'othering', are evident today in discourses about the 'dependency culture'.
- In affluent societies, relative definitions of poverty are more useful that absolute or subsistence definitions, because they are concerned with whether people have the resources to be able to participate in customary social life.
- Social workers often work with people who seem trapped in a 'cycle of deprivation'. This is better understood as a response to deprivation and disadvantage than as a primary cause of it. To do otherwise is to risk pathologizing poor people, blaming them for their own poverty.
- That the extent of poverty tends to change with socio-economic conditions strongly suggests that the main causes of poverty are structural, a product of unequal social and economic social structures. That people's chances of both becoming poor and escaping from poverty are greatly influenced by social divisions of class, 'race', gender and disability also lends weight to structural theories.
- Despite being robbed of status and autonomy by structural disadvantages, people living in poverty exercise agency to cope with and gain some control of their situation. Supporting this is a key aspect of anti-poverty practice.
- A life-course perspective can shed light on how the interaction of agency and structure can affect services users' movements in and out of poverty over time and the cumulative impact poverty can have on their health and wellbeing.

Further reading by topic

Social work and poverty

Parrott, L. (2014) *Social Work and Poverty: a critical approach*, Bristol: Policy Press

Poverty: definitions, measures and causes

Alcock, P. (2006) *Understanding Poverty*, 3rd edn, Basingstoke: Palgrave Macmillan
Holman, R. (1978) *Poverty: Explanations of Social Deprivation*, Oxford: Martin Robertson
Townsend, P. (1979) *Poverty in the United Kingdom: a survey of household resources and standards of living*, Harmondsworth: Penguin, available at: www.poverty.ac.uk/free-resources-books/poverty-united-kingdom.

'Othering', agency and the 'low-pay, no-pay cycle'

Lister, R. (2004) *Poverty*, Cambridge: Polity Press
Shildrick, T., MacDonald, Webster C. and Garthwaite, K. (2012) *Poverty and Insecurity: life in low-pay, no-pay Britain*, Bristol: Policy Press

Useful websites

Joseph Rowntree Foundation: www.jrf.org.uk

Poverty and Social Exclusion: www.poverty.ac.uk, for the 2012 consensual ('Bread-line Britain') poverty survey see the *Poverty and Social Exclusion* website at www.poverty.ac.uk/pse-research.

Social Care Institute for Excellence (SCIE) e-learning resource: *Poverty, Parenting and Social Exclusion:* www.scie.org.uk/publications/elearning/poverty/index.asp

3 Understanding social exclusion

Key messages

- Social exclusion as a concept is useful for understanding how different forms of inequality and deprivation interact over time to increase service users' social isolation and poverty.
- Different discourses of social exclusion (how it is discussed and thought about) reflect competing views about why people are excluded and what should be done about it.
- The high rates of poverty and social exclusion experienced by most ethnic minority groups are caused by the interaction of different socio-economic factors including racism.
- To tackle the social exclusion of disabled people, practice should be based on the social model of disability because it emphasizes the social causes of disability and in doing so is empowering for service users.

This chapter examines the concept of social exclusion as a way of understanding how, in an unequal society, poor and disadvantaged people are cut off from what is generally taken to be normal life. A key aspect of social exclusion is that it is multi-dimensional – excluded people are disadvantaged in many different areas of their lives. It is also a cumulative process – different forms of exclusion overlap and combine over time to increase isolation and deprivation. This is discussed in relation to ethnic minorities and disabled people, partly to show the close relationship between poverty and social exclusion. An important aspect of social exclusion is that ideas and prejudices, how we think about and therefore treat disadvantaged people, can themselves be exclusionary. An example of this, the 'ethnic poverty penalty', the 'unexplained' part of the disproportionately high rate of poverty experienced by some BME groups is discussed, to argue that this is caused by racism. Turning to examine how social workers can tackle social exclusion in practice, the importance of the social model of disability is examined. Both points, about racism and the social model of disability, may seem fairly self-evident. In fact, neither are as straightforward as they might first appear.

This chapter begins with a review of the debate about whether an 'underclass' emerged in Britain in the wake of social and economic changes in the 1980s. The underclass was presented as living separate and poorer lives than most of society. Social exclusion, which gained prominence in social policy during the Labour government of 1997 to 2010, is a different approach to similar issues: poor people and deprived areas being excluded from mainstream society and not having what most of us take for granted. A central issue here is causation: why are people excluded? The chapter applies the two theoretical approaches discussed in Chapter 2: pathological perspectives which hold that people cause their own exclusion, as compared to structural perspectives which see the primary causes as societal.

The underclass debate

Attempts to explain the riots that shook English cities in the summer of 2011 frequently invoked earlier debates about the underclass. Most explicitly, Ken Clarke, then Secretary of State for Justice, spoke of a 'sense that the hardcore of rioters came from a feral underclass, cut off from the mainstream in everything but its materialism'. Nearly 20 years earlier Clarke, then Home Secretary, had made a very similar statement deploring excuses being made 'for a section of the population who are essentially nasty pieces of work' (Clarke, 1993, quoted in Jones and Novak, 1999: 11).

Clarke's earlier outburst was part of a storm of outrage over the killing of 2-year-old Jamie Bulger by two 10-year-old boys. In the moral panic that followed, the boys' crime was depicted as a consequence of their social environment, 'a world of social and economic deprivation, of trashy television and cultural poverty, inadequate social services, failed schooling and general confusion' (Gillan, 2000). The furore had a pronounced moralistic tone, exemplified in Prime Minister John Major's injunction 'to condemn a little more and to understand a little less' (quoted in Jones and Novak, 1999: 1). Tony Blair, the future Labour Prime Minister, gained extensive coverage for a speech in which he claimed the murder was symptomatic of social and community breakdown: 'in almost any city, town or village more minor versions of the same events are becoming an almost everyday part of our lives. These are the ugly manifestations of a society which is becoming almost unworthy of the name' (quoted in Blair, 2010: 57).

This alarmism echoed reporting of the murder which, in Blair's words, 'was laced with descriptions of the life, times and mores of certain groups of young people whose families seemed separated from the mainstream' (Blair, 2010: 57). Even if the term was not always explicitly used, these accounts invoked the underclass by:

1 Focusing on a section of the poorest in society, mostly young people, who were seen as cut off from the mainstream.
2 Claiming these people lived their lives according to a different, deviant, morality than the rest of us.

In Britain 'the underclass debate' first erupted in 1989 when Charles Murray, an American political scientist who had bemoaned the growth of an underclass in the USA, was invited to the UK to investigate whether something similar was happening here. Sure enough Murray found that there was an emerging underclass: 'a growing population of working-aged, healthy people who live in a different world from other Britons, who are raising their children to live in it, and whose values are now contaminating the life of entire neighbourhoods' (Murray, 1989: 26).

For Murray this underclass had three defining characteristics: 'illegitimacy' by which he meant women having children despite not being married, violent crime and 'drop-out from the labour force'. The last of these referred not simply to high levels of youth unemployment but to 'large numbers' of young men who were physically able to work but who chose not to (Murray 1989). The significance of these three characteristics is not only that they were all said to be on the rise but also that they involved choice: young women choosing to have babies outside of marriage, for example. These choices, according to Murray, were informed by morality; the underclass was separate from the rest of us not only because they were materially worse off but also because they had different values and so behaved differently. There was then an explicit moral dimension to Murray's argument: the behaviour of the underclass was not only different, it was also wrong, even 'deplorable' (Murray, 1990: 83). Murray's analysis takes a pathological perspective, clearly saying that the underclass are the cause of the problem, because of their behaviour and morality.

What do you think? 3.1: 'The importance of blame'

Two criticisms made of Murray's underclass argument were:

1 That it is was very moralistic, blaming poor people for their poverty.
2 That it was gendered – young unmarried mothers were presented as mainly responsible for the growth of the underclass.

Read the extract below and reflect on these issues using the questions that follow.

> . . . British social policy remain[s] overwhelmingly on the side of the poor youngster who fails in school, gets in trouble with the law, does not hold a job, or has a child without being able to care for it. Youths who do any of these things will find no shortage of social workers and academics prepared to make excuses to try to shield them from the consequences of their behaviour . . . The difficulty is that, by taking away responsibility – by saying, 'Because the system is to blame, it's not your fault that . . .' – society also takes away the credit that is an essential part of the reward structure that fosters social and economic mobility.
>
> . . . I do want to reintroduce the notion of genuine blame in a moral sense . . . If one of my daughters, single and without the resources to raise a child on her own, comes home pregnant, I am not obliged to throw her out of the house. But I will think what she did is wrong . . . I will tell her so. I will love her, help her, and think hard thoughts about the male who collaborated, and find fault with myself as a father . . . but none of that will change the underlying reaction that is in my view essential for the sustenance of a civilized society. I will blame her.
>
> (Murray, 1990: 86–7)

Questions for discussion

1 Do you think Murray gives a fair representation of how social workers work with young people?
2 If, like Murray's notional daughter, poor people make 'wrong' choices, should social workers blame them for doing so?

Comment

In the extract Murray caricatures social workers. Locating people's behaviour in its social context is essential to anti-oppressive practice. As discussed in Chapter 4, teenage young women who 'come home pregnant' often make a conscious decision to have a child because it is a positive choice for them. Murray's 'civilized society' is a largely middle-class world from which they are excluded. In such circumstances, to engage in blaming, regardless of the context, risks jeopardizing any trust the teenager may have in a social worker and could be disempowering, undermining their confidence. That poor and excluded people's options are usually very limited is one reason why being non-judgemental is so important.

Murray was not the only commentator to argue that by the end of the 1980s an underclass had developed. The Labour MP and anti-poverty campaigner, Frank Field, had identified similar social groups who were cut off from society. Field's underclass consisted of three main groups: single parents, the long-term unemployed and 'elderly pensioners' (Field 1989). Field was careful to warn against over-generalizing, pointing out that in any of these groups individuals' 'attitudes and well-being will vary according to their psychological make-up and their interaction with their social environment'. But where he most clearly differed from Murray was in his analysis of why an underclass had emerged. Field identified four main causes: the rise in unemployment, widening class divisions, that those in poverty were excluded from generally rising living standards and a shift in public attitudes away from altruism and towards self-interest. For Field, what had caused an underclass to emerge were the socio-economic changes which occurred under Margaret Thatcher's Conservative government in the 1980s. In terms of blame, Field was categorical: the underclass were victims of 'a subtle form of political, social and economic apartheid' (Field, 1989: 4). In this analysis then, the causes were structural, a consequence of wider social change, and this gave Field's argument a very different emphasis from Murray's.

Social exclusion

As the 1990s progressed, policy debates about the underclass gave way to discussion of social exclusion. There were several reasons for this. While Murray's claims made for good newspaper headlines they struggled to gain academic credibility, not least because, as critics pointed out, there was scant evidence to show that a separate underclass existed (see e.g. Walker, 1990). When New Labour won the 1997 general election Blair, as Prime Minister, quickly created a Social Exclusion Unit (SEU) located in the Cabinet Office, with a brief to develop 'joined-up solutions to joined-up problems' (SEU, 2001). The rationale for this approach was that as social exclusion was seen as a multi-dimensional problem, addressing it required a coordinated response, both at a policy level (across government departments, etc.) and in practice, with local agencies and professionals working together. This raises the question of what social exclusion actually *is*. The government adopted the following, much quoted, definition: 'Social exclusion is a shorthand term for what can happen when people or areas suffer from a combination of linked problems such as unemployment, poor skills, low incomes, poor housing, high crime, bad health and family breakdown' (SEU, 2001: 10). The term 'discourse' is used a lot in the literature on social exclusion, especially in Ruth Levitas' (2005) 'three discourses of social exclusion'. Levitas uses the concept to analyse 'the language, politics and policies of New Labour' (Byrne, 2005: 54) where a discourse is 'a set of interrelated concepts', 'a matrix', which shapes understanding of social issues (Levitas, 2005: 3). In other words, discourse means the language and terminology in which the policy debate about social exclusion is conducted, including the way it is defined and how people think about it. Discourses are contested and fluid, they change over time and they reflect different social interests. The underclass debate can be seen in this way, as an argument about different understandings of social change and what should be done about it. In this debate the language used played a significant part, most starkly in Murray's use of value-laden terms such as 'illegitimate' and more recently in Clarke's 'feral underclass'. Social workers should be aware of discourses and how they influence what we think about social issues, and that they also 'constitute ways of acting in the world' (Levitas, 2005: 3). How we understand and talk about poverty and social exclusion will influence how we respond to it in practice.

What do you think? 3.2: The discourse of 'Troubled Families'

'Troubled Families' is the coalition government's flagship family intervention programme, targeted at some of the most excluded families in England. There are estimated to be 120,000 of these families, based on 2007 research which estimated that this was the number of families each of which had at least five of the following seven criteria:

No parent in the family is in work;

Family lives in overcrowded housing;

No parent has any qualifications;

Mother has mental health problems;

At least one parent has a long-standing limiting illness, disability or infirmity;

Family has low income (below 60% of median income);

Family cannot afford a number of food and clothing items.

(Levitas, 2012b: 5)

At the launch of the programme Prime Minister David Cameron said:

. . . I want to talk about troubled families. Let me be clear what I mean by this phrase. Officialdom might call them 'families with multiple disadvantages'. Some in the press might call them 'neighbours from hell'. Whatever you call them, we've known for years that a relatively small number of families are the source of a large proportion of the problems in society. Drug addiction. Alcohol abuse. Crime. A culture of disruption and irresponsibility that cascades through generations.

(Quoted in Levitas, 2012b: 6)

Questions for discussion

1 How does Cameron's description of troubled families compare to the seven criteria by which the 120,000 excluded families were originally identified?

2 What do you think the changed discourse about troubled families implies for how they are perceived in public opinion and how services should respond to them?

Comment

The seven aspects of social exclusion emphasize poverty with related problems like poor health and bad housing. They do not explicitly address causes but could perhaps by implication be read as leaning towards the causes of poverty and social exclusion being structural. Cameron, by contrast, emphasizes characteristics which are much more likely to be seen as pathological (substance abuse and crime) and claims these families are not only to blame for their own problems but also that they are the 'source of a large proportion of the problems in society'.

The shift is striking (for a full analysis see Levitas, 2012b). What Cameron and his government have promoted is a discourse which:

1 Portrays troubled families as pathological and undeserving, emblematic of the dependency culture which their welfare reform strategy seeks to eradicate.
2 Is very reminiscent of Murray's underclass thesis.

This discourse is clearly not intended to win public sympathy for the families concerned. As social workers are in the forefront of local implementation of the Troubled Families programme it is important both to be aware of such discourses and not to let one's judgement and values be swayed by them.

Levitas' three discourses of social exclusion are RED, MUD and SID, where RED is redistribution discourse, MUD a moral underclass discourse and SID a social integrationist one. As Levitas says in summarizing the discourses, in all of them paid work is seen as a key route out of exclusion and all have a moral content. As a shorthand, and 'oversimplified', way of distinguishing them, focusing on what excluded people are thought to lack can be useful: 'in RED they have no money, in SID they have no work, in MUD they have no morals' (Levitas, 2005: 27). With each discourse, the solution to the problems flows from what is thought to be lacking:

In RED, the assumption is that the resources available in cash and kind to the poor need to be increased both relatively and absolutely, implying both improved levels of income maintenance and better access to public and private services. In SID the solution is increasing labour market participation, for paid work is claimed to deliver inclusion, both directly and indirectly through the income it provides. In MUD, the emphasis is on changing behaviour through a mixture of carrots and sticks – manipulation of welfare benefits, sanctions for non-compliance [now called 'conditionality'] and intensive social work with individuals.

(Levitas, 2005: x)

Another way of distinguishing between Levitas' discourses is that RED is broad in its approach, seeing exclusion as a product of general social processes whereas SID and, especially, MUD, have a much narrower focus on excluded people as 'the problem'.

Social exclusion is complex – there are many dimensions to it and many manifestations of it; accordingly definitions have to be general and cannot specify all the causes
and forms. That said, one of the 'stronger' definitions is:

> Social exclusion is a complex and multi-dimensional process. It involves the
> lack or denial of resources, rights, goods and services, and the inability to par-
> ticipate in the normal relationships and activities, available to the majority of
> people in a society, whether in economic, social, cultural or political arenas. It
> affects both the quality of life of individuals and the equity and cohesion of soci-
> ety as a whole.
>
> (Levitas *et al.*, 2007: 25)

The strengths of this definition are that it locates both the causes and consequences of
exclusion in their general social context, sees it as a process rather than a static condition
and, in the reference to 'denial', acknowledges that social exclusion is something that is
done *to* people (by other people), it is not a byproduct of amorphous processes over
which we have no control. For these reasons it fits well with social work theories, values
and practice.

Neighbourhood effects

Another important aspect of social exclusion is that it can be related to areas, or neighbourhoods. Concern about deprived areas, especially what Tony Blair called 'no go/no
exit' areas was a major factor in the setting up of the SEU in 1997. In 2010, when the
newly formed coalition government reviewed the *State of the Nation* they found 'whole
communities existing on the margins of society' (Cabinet Office, 2010: 3). On one level,
deprived areas can be seen as places, neighbourhoods, estates, etc., where there are concentrations of poor people. The *State of the Nation*, for example, says that half of all
children in families living on benefits lived in the 20 per cent of most deprived neighbourhoods. One implication of this is that conditions in these areas are likely to be much
worse than in society generally. One authoritative report on economic inequality found
that 'The differences between people living in the poorest and richest areas are some of
the most dramatic that our work reveals ... some of the differences are startling'
(National Equality Panel, 2010: 249). Stark differences in educational attainment, employment, income and wealth are both a cause and consequence of sharp inequalities in life
chances. Perhaps the most brutal form this takes is that people in poor areas live shorter
lives: they are on average likely to die seven years earlier than people in the richest areas
(Marmot Review Team, 2010).

But the characteristics of deprived areas can be more than just an aggregate of the
disadvantage of the people who live in them: there might be additional 'neighbourhood
effects'. Lupton and Kneale (2010: 7) define this as:

> effects arising from characteristics of the neighbourhood, whether these are
> demographic, social, physical or institutional: the idea being that the area exerts
> an influence, over and above any individual characteristics. If there are neigh-
> bourhood effects, similar people living in different neighbourhoods will have
> different outcomes.

In 2010 there were some 5 million people living in the 10 per cent most deprived areas of England (Department for Communities and Local Government, 2011). The implication of area effects is that for these people, their social exclusion will be deepened by the characteristics of the neighbourhoods in which they live.

How neighbourhood affects work and their significance is much debated. But there is compelling evidence to show that the characteristics of localities can make a difference to poor people's lives. That some forms of child abuse, particularly neglect, are linked to poverty is well established (Dyson, 2008). However, Gordon Jack (2004) argues that this can be exacerbated by the areas in which they live: 'the actual stresses experienced by parents, levels of child abuse and various aspects of children's behaviour and development have all been shown to vary between apparently similar neighbourhoods and communities' (p. 374). Jack estimates local area effects are significant, 'accounting for something like 20–25 per cent of the differences found [between areas]'. While Ghate and Hazel's (2002) research on the impact of 'poor environments' on parenting generally found that it was difficult to separate out the effects of individual- from area-level poverty, they concluded that 'living in a poor area clearly does contribute independently of other factors to parenting stress'(p. 103). The main risk factors of poor areas that parents identified were feeling oppressed by fear of crime, local environmental hazards (e.g. dog mess) being perceived as a threat to their families and, for some, feelings of isolation due to high population turnover. The poorer the areas were, the worse the neighbourhood effects were.

Teenage pregnancy and parenthood is also associated with poverty and social exclusion: teenage girls/women who are poor are more likely to become pregnant and they and their children are much more likely to experience various forms of social exclusion subsequently. The Labour government's Teenage Pregnancy Strategy, introduced in 1999, was based on the assumption that because there were geographic concentrations of teenage pregnancy, neighbourhood effects were a factor in the UK having the 'worst record on teenage pregnancies in Europe' (SEU, 1999: 4). Lupton and Kneale (2010: 14) however, found that the statistical evidence to support this policy was inconclusive but, looking at qualitative studies on teenage pregnancy they concluded that '. . . neighbourhood and wider area influences might be associated with an early planned (or anticipated) pregnancy and with the propensity and opportunity to engage in risky sexual behaviour leading to unplanned pregnancy'.

One practice implication of this is that, while it might be hard to quantify, at what might be called a common-sense level there seems little doubt that social exclusion (and poverty) can be worsened by local conditions and practical experience of working in and with local communities can give valuable insights into how this happens. Hence Lupton and Kneale's call for 'practitioner knowledge' to be used to inform policy-making. Working with communities to tackle poverty and social exclusion is discussed in Chapter 8; here though, Spicker's (2007: 40) unequivocal answer to the question as to can neighbourhoods 'make poverty worse' is worth noting: 'People who live in particular areas are more likely than people in other areas to be poor as a consequence of the place where they live . . . [thus] the answer has to be "yes".'

The existence of neighbourhood effects, however difficult they are to measure, does suggest that the main causes of social exclusion are structural. The most useful, or strongest, definitions of social exclusion do the same. While the pathologizing legacy of Murray's underclass lives on in the MUD discourse, an advantage of conceiving of multiple disadvantage and inequality as social exclusion is that it can be used to focus on structural causes.

Ethnic minorities and social exclusion

A feature of the post-Second World War growth of the ethnic minority population in the UK was their concentration in urban areas, mainly Greater London, the West Midlands, Greater Manchester and West Yorkshire. As Harrison (with Phillips, 2003) and others have shown, this was linked to urban deprivation: reflecting their marginalization in employment and housing. BME groups were, and still are, more likely to live in 'poor areas' in inner cities. More recently, while 'new immigration' since the 1990s has in some ways followed different patterns of settlement, it is still the case that the geographic distribution of the BME population is significantly different from the white British majority and is disproportionately concentrated in deprived areas (Amas, 2008). Kenway and Palmer (2007: 21) give a useful summary of ethnic minorities' distinct but varied pattern of settlement in Great Britain:

> the proportion of the population belonging to an ethnic minority . . . [ranges] from 50 per cent and 35 per cent in inner and outer London respectively to less than 5 per cent across Wales, Scotland, the rural areas of England and the urban areas in the North East.

However, residential integration is increasing (Catney, 2013) and claims that we are 'sleepwalking to segregation' 'turn out to be myths, unsustainable in the face of evidence' (Finney and Simpson, 2009: 2). There are many factors which influence where people live but it is a truism of poor areas that people who have the means to do so are likely to move out (Fenton *et al.*, 2010). There is evidence that the Asian population is becoming more dispersed, but those of Indian origin are 'much more likely to move up the housing ladder' than Pakistanis or Bangladeshis (Beider and Netto, 2012). That the latter two groups have the highest poverty rates of all ethnic minority groups (see below) is a factor in this.

For all the variations and changes it remains the case that ethnic minorities are over-represented in deprived areas. This is one of many forms of disadvantage which BME groups suffer; it can be useful for social workers to think about such disadvantage as social exclusion because doing so can show how prejudice, inequality and poverty impact on people's lives in ways that are both systematic and cumulative: they do not happen by chance and their overall effect on people's life chances is huge.

One immediately striking fact is the scale of poverty among ethnic minorities, especially when compared to that of the white British majority. For ethnic minority groups as a whole the poverty rate was about 40 per cent in 2003–5; this was about twice the rate for the white majority. However, for some groups the rates are higher: 65 per cent for Bangladeshis, 55 per cent for Pakistanis and 45 per cent for Black Africans (Kenway and Palmer, 2007). To put it more starkly, two thirds of Bangladeshis live in income poverty – three times the proportion for White British people.

As we have seen, poverty is a major determinant of people's life chances so these figures are indicative of the extent of wider inequalities in British society. That over half of Bangladeshi and Pakistani children 'can expect to be growing up in poverty' (Platt, 2009: 25) is a fact that will probably follow them across their life course, with consequences for their wellbeing.

The high levels of poverty experienced by ethnic minority groups is a major factor in, and cause of their social exclusion. However, the nature of poverty among BME communities is complex; while it is possible to identify common features between ethnic minority groups there is also great variation within and between them. Two concepts which are useful for understanding this complexity are 'intersectionality' and the 'ethnic poverty penalty'.

Intersectionality

Social exclusion is multi-dimensional because it reflects the diversity and complexity of people's lives. The statistics cited above show clearly that ethnicity is a major risk factor for poverty. But other factors – for example, gender, age, religion, disability, class and where you live – will also influence your chances of being poor. Intersectionality is the recognition of the multiplicity of factors which can affect people's life chances and thus which need to be taken into account in anti-poverty work. Barnard and Turner (2011: 4) give an example to illustrate this:

> The experience of a middle class, third generation, Indian, Hindu woman with a degree, living in Milton Keynes may have little in common with a second generation, Indian, Muslim woman, with a level three qualification, living in Bradford with a disabled husband and two children.

The two women have similar ethnicity in that their families both come from India, but their lives, and the likelihood of them being poor and excluded, are very different. Intersectionality helps in understanding poverty and exclusion because it can shed light on the interaction of two general factors. First is what Barnard and Turner (2011: 4) call 'the centrality of informal processes in shaping poverty outcomes: the texture of day-to-day life, the decisions and assumptions that people make'. The second factor is the general social structures which shape and constrain these decisions. In a study of Bangladeshi, Pakistani and black Caribbean women's employment the Equal Opportunities Commission (2007) found that this is affected not only by ethnicity and gender but also by geography – for example, in Croydon 45 per cent of Pakistani women are economically active but in Cardiff only 26 per cent are. This wide variation will be influenced by many things but the local labour market will clearly be a major determinant of what job opportunities are available to ethnic minority women. Intersectionality should not be used to discount the significance of either ethnicity or racism but can enhance understanding of how they affect outcomes for different people in different situations. It can also help practitioners avoid making assumptions based on stereotypes about ethnic minority groups.

The ethnic poverty penalty

The concept of an ethnic penalty has been used to denote how much of the greater poverty of ethnic minority groups cannot be explained by variations in known or observable risk factors. We do know, for example, that children in single-parent households and large families are at greater risk of poverty. We also know that about half of all Black Caribbean and Black African households are single-parent families, twice the rate of the White British majority; and that about two thirds of Pakistani and Bangladeshi families have three or more children, again twice the rate of the White British majority (Platt, 2009). However, as Lucinda Platt has shown, such differences in family composition and other risk factors only go part of the way to explaining ethnic minorities' higher poverty rates. Put simply, the part that is not explained is the 'poverty penalty'.

But the impact or significance of risk factors varies between ethnic groups. Platt (2009) explains, for instance, that while children in single-parent families, as compared to families with two parents, are more likely to be poor in most ethnic groups (White British,

Indian, Black Caribbean and Black African) this does not hold for all groups: Pakistani and Bangladeshi children face a greater of risk of poverty if they are in two-parent families. A further aspect is how risk factors combine. About half of Black African families are single parent households and about half have three or more children. As Platt suggests, these two types of family probably overlap (i.e. a relatively high proportion of Black African children probably live in large, one-parent families) which helps to explain why Black African single-parent families are at greater risk of poverty than the average. There are other risk factors, of course. Platt looks at households by employment status, income and the number of adults by health/disability status. While these factors all play a part, she concludes that 'we cannot understand ethnic group differences in child poverty in terms of variations in particular family and household characteristics alone' (Platt, 2009: 35). An important implication of this is that targeting interventions on particular household types – for example, single parents, will not resolve the problem of ethnic minorities' higher rates of poverty. As Platt says, the difference will remain, the difference being the ethnic poverty penalty.

Gender is also a factor: ethnic minority women are, as Moosa (with Woodroffe, 2009) says, more likely to be poor than ethnic minority men and white British women. This is partly because employment rates are lower; in 2008 nearly three quarters (72.6 per cent) of white British women were in paid work compared to little more than a quarter of Pakistani and Bangladeshi women (25.4 and 28.1 per cent respectively). Ethnic minority women who have jobs face a range of associated disadvantages: they are more likely to be in low-paid, insecure and part-time work with fewer benefits. Although employment rates vary between groups, ethnic minority women who do work are more likely to be mothers than their white British counterparts. These women are, to varying extents, caught between two pincers. On one side they generally have less access to childcare and pay more for what they do have (Craig, 2005); on the other side, child-friendly, flexible employment is harder to find. Black mothers, in particular, are more likely to be lone parents and working but have 'the lowest level of access to flexible working arrangements' (Moosa with Woodroffe, 2009: 18). All of this can be related to the ethnic poverty penalty. Research shows, for example, that despite their generally disadvantaged position in the labour market, employed Bangladeshi, Pakistani and black Caribbean women are more likely to have a degree than working white British women (Equal Opportunities Commission, 2007).

It is a complex issue, an example of intersectionality: employment, gender, family and household structure, culture and other factors all influence ethnic minorities' higher poverty rates. Nonetheless, there is clear evidence of an ethnic poverty penalty: something else 'unexplained'. For social workers, what causes this penalty is a crucial question, not least in the immediate practical sense that if we want to address service users' poverty we need to understand its causes. This, of course, is linked to the ethical commitment to challenge social injustice. The obvious issue here is racism. In discussing the ethnic penalty in (male) employment, Emejulu (2008: 165) is unequivocal: 'There can be no escaping the fact that endemic racism is the cause of the systematic disadvantage of these groups . . .'. Platt (2009: 56) is more cautious, arguing that the fact of a poverty penalty 'does not directly imply discrimination'; but she acknowledges that 'it is likely that discrimination may contribute indirectly to ethnic poverty penalties'. This seems to miss the point that racism is systematic: it affects social groups in general and pervades most, if not all, areas of social life.

In relation to poverty this can be seen at both institutional and individual levels. Law (2012) points out that all BME groups are more likely to depend on means-tested, rather than contributory, benefits than the majority White British population. There is also evidence of significant non-take up of benefits – for example, with Disability Living Allowance (DLA) Salway *et al.* (2007: 56) found that 'compared with White British respondents with comparable health and socioeconomic status, Pakistanis, Bangladeshis and Black Africans had much lower probabilities of receiving DLA'. Language barriers, stigma and lack of knowledge are among the reasons for this, but it is, nonetheless, institutional racism: the policies, procedures and practices by which benefits are made available (or not) result in ethnic minorities being excluded and impoverished. At an individual level, in job interviews young Bangladeshi, Pakistani and Black Caribbean women have been found to be two to three times more likely to be asked about their plans about marriage and having children than White British women (Equal Opportunities Commission, 2007) with obvious implications for employment.

Disability and social exclusion

In some ways the poverty and social exclusion of disabled people and their carers is similar to that of ethnic minorities, in particular:

- the extent of poverty is much greater than for the majority or for the population on average;
- the causes are complex and varied and are compounded by discrimination.

Responding to this challenges social workers to move beyond the traditional individualistic focus of practice.

By what is at the time of writing the main government measure of poverty (the 60 per cent HBAI poverty line, discussed in Chapter 2), about 30 per cent of disabled adults are poor; roughly twice the rate of poverty among non-disabled adults (Palmer, 2006). In 2011 some 10 million people reported having a limiting illness or disability (ONS, 2013b); so it follows that about 3.3 million of these were poor by the HBAI measure. Yet this is a significant underestimate because the HBAI poverty line, being based on income, fails to take account of the higher costs of living faced by disabled people. Disabled people report facing extra costs in most areas of everyday life. These additional costs increase with need and they also affect carers. The income of disabled people living on benefits was estimated (c. 2004) to be £200 per week below what they needed to have 'an acceptable, equitable quality of life' (Smith *et al.*, 2004). Disabled adults are more likely to be reliant on benefits because they are less likely to be in work. And those who are employed earn less than similarly qualified non-disabled people are likely to earn (Disability Alliance, 2010).

Inevitably poverty such as this is linked to social exclusion, with disabled people being unable to participate in things which are taken for granted or appear normal for most people; as disabled people themselves testify:

> I don't do paid work but was doing voluntary work but have been resigning from committees because I just can't cope. This is my precious tenuous link with my community going up the spout.
>
> (Alannah)

> Many activities I would like to attend are at weekends and I only have help getting up on weekdays, so I miss such concerts, festivals etc.
>
> (Geoff, quoted in Brawn *et al.*, 2013: 32)

It can also be demeaning – and devastating:

> My repeated failure to obtain due support ... has made me feel rejected,
> excluded, worthless, irrelevant and of no value to society. The resultant abys-
> mally poor quality of life and standard of living I have to endure has caused me
> permanent damage and injury to my wellbeing, over and above the injuries sus-
> tained through no fault of my own ... I have lost much of my self-respect and
> confidence.
>
> (Martin quoted in Brawn *et al.*, 2013: 38)

One response to people in such difficulties can be to see them as 'personal tragedies':
the unfortunate but apparently random visitation of disadvantage. This is a mistake
social workers should avoid. The onset of disability is linked to age: most people who
become disabled do so when they are adults and the risks increase with age; for older
people illness and accidents are more likely to result in disability. However, as Burchardt
(2003) has shown there is a clear socio-economic gradient in the onset of disability – for
instance, adults with no educational qualifications are four times more likely to become
disabled than those with degrees. In terms of income distribution, adults in the bottom
20 per cent (the poorest fifth, or quintile, of the population) are two and a half times more
likely to become disabled than people in the top 20 per cent. There is also a clear North-
South divide (in England). The 2011 census found the widest regional variation was
between the North East, where 21.6 per cent reported a limiting long-term illness or disability, and London, where 14.2 per cent did (ONS, 2013b). The chances of being disabled,
and excluded, are then not random but are systematically distributed in relation to
socio-economic status. They are a manifestation of the social inequalities in health discussed in Chapter 4. And these inequalities are significant: the 'health gap' measured in
years spent free of disability is wider than that for life expectancy (Marmot Review
Team, 2010).

There is also a two-way relationship between disability and social inequalities or, as
Burchardt (2003: 62) puts it: 'someone who is socially excluded is at greater risk of
becoming disabled, and someone who becomes disabled is at greater risk of becoming
socially excluded'. This fact can help clarify arguments about pathological and structural
causes of poverty and exclusion. While pathological perspectives usually involve some
element of victim-blaming, the personal tragedy view is similar in that it focuses on individuals albeit with more sympathy than is usually given to poor people. Yet the overwhelming evidence about the systematic link between disability and other forms of social
disadvantage points strongly towards a structural explanation. Much the same can
be said of the poverty and hardship that many of the 6.4 million unpaid carers endure
(Carers UK, 2011).

A structural perspective on the poverty and exclusion of disabled people is complementary to the social model of disability: a way of understanding the societal causes of
disability. The social model of disability developed by the Disabled People's Movement:
disabled people coming together to struggle for equality and civil rights from the early
1970s (Oliver, 2009). It directly challenges the individual model and the related medicalization of disability which have dominated policy and services. The fundamental flaw of
the individual model is in the name: it locates the problem with individuals: 'there's something wrong with them' (Oliver, 2009: 44). This lends itself to medicalization, seeing disability as a physical or biological 'problem' to be addressed by medical intervention. The
social model challenges this by drawing a sharp distinction between impairment and
disability where:

Impairment is a condition of the body or mind, such as lacking a limb, being partially sighted, or experiencing depression. It is an attribute of an individual. Disability is the loss or limitation of opportunities to take part in the life of the community on an equal level with others. It arises from the social, economic and physical environment in which people with impairments find themselves.

(Burchardt, 2003: 736)

A related distinction is between illness and disability. This is crucial to the social model because, as Oliver explains, 'Most illnesses are treatable and even curable by medical interventions; most impairments are not curable; and all disability can be eradicated by change to the way we organize society' (2009: 44). With the shift of focus in how disability is understood there is also a change in who is seen as having an active, central role in overcoming disability. As might be expected of a perspective developed by and for disabled people, the social model is empowering:

[It] offers a way to organise politically against the principles of social and economic exclusion, and oppression in a disabilist society. It gives a critique of all that has gone before based on individualism and the market. It also argues that disabled people must be at the centre of voicing their own experiences.

(Jolly, 2012: 3)

The social model emphasizes the ways in which people with impairments are socially excluded by the disabling barriers society puts in their way:

These barriers include inaccessible education, information and communication systems, working environments, inadequate disability benefits, discriminatory health and social support services, inaccessible transport, housing and public buildings and amenities, and the devaluing of people labelled 'disabled' by negative imagery and representation in the media – films, television and newspapers.

(Barnes, 2004: 5)

This is evident in the accounts of parents of disabled children (quoted in Preston, 2005: 20) describing some of the routine things which their families miss out on:

. . . trips to the cinema, swimming pool and other leisure activities. Eating out together is impossible, eating together in our own home is a nightmare, which means there is no way we could have friends round for a meal.

(Anon.)

. . . joining clubs, going on proper holidays, being able to access play schemes during the holiday, as child 2 is severely disabled he cannot access a vast range of activities without constant supervision, bike rides, days out to theme parks, going out for meals, birthday parties, picnics, staying over at friend's houses, not having to plan each to military precision.

(Anon.)

Barnes (2004: 5) summarizes the social model as 'nothing more complicated than an emphasis on the economic, environmental and cultural barriers encountered by people viewed by others as having some form of impairment'. As such it can help social workers avoid the inherent tendency in individualist/casework methodologies to pathologize service users.

In campaigning on and for the social model the Disabled People's Movement has won significant reforms including anti-discriminatory legislation, social security benefits (in particular DLA) and direct payments (for a list see Jolly, 2012). Self-directed support and personalization also originated with the Disabled People's Movement, based on social model principles (Beresford, 2009). What began as an explicit challenge to, and rejection of, orthodox policy and practice has become mainstream, now almost universally endorsed by policy-makers and service providers. This success has brought problems, one being incorporation. Universal endorsement of the social model often comes 'without any substantial changes in practices' by service providers (Oliver and Barnes, 2012). More specifically, both Morris (2011) and Jolly (2012) argue that the coalition government (and New Labour before it) pays lip-service to the social model while in practice imposing a regime which is informed by a bio-psycho-social model. The latter is, they argue, essentially a development of the individual model which acknowledges the psychological and social aspects of illness as well as the medical/biological. This is progress but the model, they claim, remains focused on individuals as the problem and the distinction between impairment and disability is absent. In this sense the model is reactionary; Jolly (2012: 1) for instance points out that the model 'ridiculously claims that we can think ourselves out of being disabled'.

These conflicting theories about how disability is understood might seem abstract and academic. But if proof were needed that theory matters, the coalition government's enforcement of the Work Capability Assessment amply provides it. The Work Capacity Assessment is used to determine whether people are too ill or disabled to work – and therefore whether they are eligible for Employment and Support Allowance (ESA) or Job Seekers' Allowance (JSA), which is lower and to get it claimants have to actively seek work. People who are too sick or disabled to work are the largest group of claimants of out of work benefits, numbering some 2.6 million in 2010 (Palmer, 2011). But governments (coalition and New Labour) assume that many of these people are not really ill or impaired so should be in work (Morris, 2011). It is, in some politicians' eyes, a manifestation of the 'dependency culture'. Hence the coalition government's aims to reduce by 1 million the number of people claiming sickness-related benefits. The Work Capability Assessment is the means by which it hopes to do this.

The Work Capability Assessment has been widely criticized on two grounds. One is that it is unduly harsh and does not take account of the reality of living with an impairment. Here a much-cited figure is that 38 per cent of appeals against Work Capability Assessment decisions are upheld. A House of Commons review noted that this poor decision-making 'caused claimants considerable distress' particularly for the most vulnerable ones. The review concluded that 'The standardised "tick-box" approach fails to adequately account for rare, variable or mental health conditions and this can lead to greater inaccuracies in decision-making for these particular claimant groups' (Public Accounts Committee, 2013: 3). This has probably been the main or most publicized type of criticism, that the Work Capability Assessment is unfair: too rigid, too harsh and so causing unnecessary hardship to claimants put through the process. The recommended solution that follows from this analysis is to make the Work Capability Assessment fairer. The Hardest Hit coalition, for example, call for reform of the Work Capability Assessment, to take more account of the complexity of disabled people's lives and to give claimants better information (Kaye et al., 2012). A weakness of this approach is that it can reflect an implicit acceptance of the underlying philosophy of the Work Capability Assessment: an individual/medical model of disability. The perceived problem is not in the well documented ways that disabled people are disadvantaged in, and denied access to, employment (see e.g. Preston, 2006). Rather it is seen to lie with individuals who must be 'encouraged' to seek work by being put through the assessment process.

There is a tragic irony in this given that it is happening in the midst of an economic downturn characterized by high levels of unemployment and underemployment. The tragedy is in the suffering inflicted on the people being assessed. Evidence of the stress, illness and hardship the Work Capability Assessment has caused is extensive; particularly powerful is *The People's Review of the Work Capability Assessment* (Spartacus, 2012) which shows that it has also cost people their lives. Another irony is that while the government presents work as the best route out of poverty, the Work Capability Assessment and related reforms are creating exclusion. One survey found that 84 per cent of disabled people feared that losing DLA 'would drive them into isolation and struggling to manage their condition' (Kaye *et al.*, 2012: 9).

What do you think? 3.3: Disability and discourses of exclusion

Commenting on 2011 figures which suggested that 'only one in four' ESA claimants could not work, Prime Minister David Cameron claimed that:

> For too long in this country we have left people on welfare for year after year when those people, with help and with assistance, could work, and so we're producing a much better system where we really put people through their paces and say that if you can work, you should work . . . That will be good for them, good for their families and good for our economy.
>
> (Quoted in Wintour, 2011)

Questions for discussion

1 Which of Levitas' discourses of social exclusion (discussed earlier) best explains the government's drive to reduce the number of people claiming disability related benefits through the Work Capability Assessment? The three discourses are: RED, the redistribution discourse; MUD, the moral underclass discourse and SID, a social integrationist one.
2 How might you explain the difference in tone between Cameron's statement and the way many disabled people experience the Work Capability Assessment?

Comment

As with much welfare reform, the Work Capability Assessment illustrates well the gap between how policy can be presented by politicians and its implementation in practice. The quote by Cameron sits comfortably within the SID discourse: by working, disabled people will be integrated into society and that is for the general good. The harsh reality of the Work Capability Assessment fits much better with the MUD discourse, where claimants are seen as deviant and the aim is to change their behaviour, to 'cure' them of 'dependency'. The gap between presentation and practice might be explained in terms of electoral politics: blaming disabled people for their social exclusion is probably not a vote-winner.

The ESA/Work Capability Assessment process is very focused on individuals. The assessment is primarily 'about identifying levels of impairment rather than experiences of disabling barriers' (Morris, 2011: 4). Likewise the 'help and assistance' for ESA claimants deemed capable of beginning to look for work immediately is to be focused on the individual and can include unpaid work experience. Thus, despite the claims about recognizing the social model of disability, the reform of benefits for disabled people is much more based on an individual or bio-psycho-social model. That the consequent failure to recognize the disabling barriers society erects has caused much hardship for disabled people might be expected.

For social workers, besides supporting disabled people in their struggles with and against welfare reform of this kind, there are also lessons to be learned about the relation between theory and practice. Although Oliver *et al.* (2012) criticize the social work profession for failing to develop an adequate theoretical understanding of disability, most social workers are probably aware of and subscribe to the social model. The difficulty is that most social work practice has 'been unable to shake loose from the individual model embedded in social consciousness generally' (Oliver *et al.*, 2012: 25). To 'shake loose' and practise within the social model requires a more collaborative and collective approach. This can be done with all of the three main social work methods: casework, group work and community work. But it involves a shift from helping individuals adapt to 'the personal disaster' of impairment, the onset of disability, to helping them identify and obtain the personal, social, financial and community resources that will enable them to participate fully in social life.

A useful illustration of how this might be approached is Burchardt's (2004) discussion of how the capabilities framework of poverty (see Chapter 2) can be used with the social model of disability. Here she compares how questions about people's experience of disability can be framed in three different ways. As Table 3.1 shows, the major difference between the three approaches is that the individual model questions are 'internal', or personal to the person being asked, while the social model and, less explicitly, the capabilities framework questions are more concerned with external, social factors. We might quibble about the wording of the questions but the aim here is not to provide a blueprint, but, rather, to suggest how in working to tackle the social exclusion of disabled people using an approach informed by the social model has several advantages, not least that:

Table 3.1 Three ways of asking about disability

Individual model	Social model	Capabilities framework
Can you tell me what is wrong with you?	Can you tell me what is wrong with society?	Compared to others, are your opportunities to do things you would like to do limited?
Does your health problem/ disability prevent you from going out as often or as far as you would like?	What is it about the local environment that makes it difficult for you to get about in your neighbourhood?	What are the constraints on your going out as often or as far as you would like?
Does your health problem/ disability make it difficult for you to travel by bus?	Are there any transport or financial problems which prevent you from going out as far or as often as you would like?	How easy is it for you to get to a destination a couple of miles from your home?

Source: adapted from Burchardt (2004, Table 1: 741)

- it avoids pathologizing people with impairments;
- it locates the barriers that cause their exclusion in the social environment in which they live;
- it provides a first step towards identifying the resources that can enable them to overcome those barriers.

Social work can make a significant contribution to overcoming the entrenched exclusion of disabled people or it can be a barrier to their inclusion. Embedding the social model in practice has the potential to allow social workers to play a progressive role in work with disabled people. The challenge for the profession is, as Sheldon and Macdonald note (2009: 334), to 'be relevant or be gone'.

Summary of main points

- The debate about whether there was an underclass in the 1990s was, in part, about competing explanations of multiple deprivation. This was taken up in the Labour government's drive to reduce social exclusion from 1997, with social exclusion being seen as resulting from the interaction of many factors: poverty, unemployment, bad housing, educational underachievement, etc. (rather than focusing only on poverty and income).
- Social exclusion takes account of the multiple ways people can be marginalized and that this can be a cumulative process, worsening over time. It also recognizes that deprivation can be concentrated in small areas with 'neighbourhood effects' worsening the poverty of the people who live in them.
- Levitas' (2005) RED, MUD and SID discourses highlight differences in accounts of the nature and causes of social exclusion; is it, at root, because people lack money, morals or work? From this follow different views about what are appropriate responses, both in policy and practice.
- The high rates of poverty of most ethnic minority groups are in part a product of the multiple disadvantages BME groups suffer in, for example, education, employment and housing.
- While social workers should be sensitive to the complex factors that can cause people from BME groups to be excluded, they should also be aware that the evidence of an 'ethnic poverty penalty' strongly suggests that racism remains a major factor in the poverty and social exclusion of BME groups.
- The social model of disability emphasizes that it is social barriers which are the main cause of the social exclusion of disabled people. Although in theory the social model is now widely accepted, policy and practice too often reflects an individual model, failing to take adequate account of structural causes.

Further reading by topic

Social exclusion

Levitas, R. (2005) *The Inclusive Society? Social exclusion and New Labour*, 2nd edn, Basingstoke: Palgrave Macmillan.
Pierson, J. (2010) *Tackling Social Exclusion*, 2nd edn, London: Routledge.

The underclass

Morris, L. (1994) *Dangerous Classes: the underclass and social citizenship*, London: Routledge

Welshman, J. (2007) *Underclass: a history of the excluded, 1880–2000*, London: Hambledon Continuum.

Ethnic minorities and social exclusion

Craig, G., Atkin, K., Chattoo, S. and Flynn, R. (eds) (2012) *Understanding 'Race' and Ethnicity: theory, history, policy, practice*, Bristol: Policy Press.

Platt, L. (2009) *Ethnicity and Child Poverty*, Research Report No. 576, London: Department for Work and Pensions.

Disability and social exclusion

Morris, J. (2011) *Rethinking Disability Policy*, York: Joseph Rowntree Foundation.

Oliver, M., Sapey, B. and Thomas, P. (2012) *Social Work with Disabled People*, Basingstoke: Palgrave Macmillan.

Useful websites

Runnymede Trust, 'the UK's leading independent race equality think-tank': www.runnymedetrust.org

The (Leeds) Disability Archive UK: www.leeds.ac.uk/disability-studies/archiveuk

We are Spartacus, 'disabled people's views on welfare reform': http://wearespartacus.org.uk/

4 Broken Britain? The social context of poverty and social exclusion

> **Key messages**
> - Poverty and social exclusion are linked to profound social changes including growing individualism, consumerism and community breakdown which, in turn, are linked to neo-liberal globalization.
> - These changes not only shape the social context of practice, they also influence social work policy and practice in, for example, care management and what Dustin (2007) calls the 'McDonaldization of social work'.
> - Most service users are affected by social inequalities in health which are caused by poverty and social exclusion. These inequalities are thus a form of social injustice with which social workers should engage.
> - High levels of social inequality are a cause of many of the social problems, such as teenage pregnancy, drug abuse and mental distress, which social workers deal with in practice.

> Social breakdown is perhaps the greatest challenge facing Britain today. The economic downturn has had a devastating impact, but the slow journey to recovery has begun. Sadly, we cannot say the same about our social recession; this will take much longer to fix.
>
> (Pickles, 2010: 161)

This statement by a Conservative Party policy advisor captures two linked themes of the 2010 general election, out of which came the Conservative-Liberal Democrat coalition government. The first theme was that, after the economic collapse of 2008, there was near universal agreement that the overriding government priority had to be restoring economic growth. The second theme was that, irrespective of the recession, there was an underlying social crisis: British society was somehow 'broken'.

The 'Broken Britain' trope has been described as 'an accordion-like concept, stretching and squeezing to fit different definitions depending on what the major worry of the hour is' (Gentleman, 2010). It does, however, have two key features:

1 A notion that there is a generalized social crisis or breakdown of some sort.
2 That poverty and social exclusion are central to that crisis (see e.g., Centre for Social Justice, 2006).

Whether or not British society is broken, there is no shortage of evidence, some of it discussed here, that there is widespread unease about recent social changes, changes which shape the context of social work practice. This chapter explores that context to suggest ways of understanding it that can usefully inform practice with people who are poor and socially excluded. The chapter begins by showing that these changes have their roots in the economic restructuring which is associated with neo-liberal globalization. The social impact of this has been vast, in particular, poverty and social exclusion have become widespread and, as has been shown in earlier chapters, this has been accompanied by historically high levels of inequality. The effects of this social inequality are discussed in relation to two issues:

1 Health inequalities as a social work issue.
2 General social inequality as a cause of many of the problems that blight service users' lives.

Recent moral panics about teenage pregnancy, parenting and poverty are used to explore these issues and their implications for practice. Understanding how poverty and inequality can affect people's lives and inform the choices they make underpins anti-oppressive practice. Moreover, the professional commitment to social justice requires a critical engagement with social inequality and the damage it inflicts on people.

The breaking of Britain?

The 'Broken Britain' refrain in 2010 echoed the general election of 1997, when poverty and social exclusion were seen as central to a perceived social crisis. The victorious Labour leader, Tony Blair, later described that crisis in the following terms:

> We had a poor record in this country in adapting to social and economic change. The result was sharp income inequality, a third of children growing up in poverty, a host of social problems such as homelessness and drug abuse, and divisions in society typified by deprived neighbourhoods that had become no go areas for some and no exit zones for others. All of us bore the cost of social breakdown – directly, or through the costs to society and the public finances.
>
> (Blair, foreword to SEU, 2001: 4)

The roots of these changes go far back but under the Thatcherite Conservative government of the 1980s, 'the sheer pace and scale of such developments . . . had the effect of transforming them from changes of degree to changes in kind' (Harris, 2009: 16). The transition to a service economy was central to this, with de-industrialization accompanying wider changes:

> . . . many aspects of British local and national culture appeared to become far less cohesive and distinctive than in any earlier period of history. This was not just because of 'modernisation', but because the closure or foreign takeover of many major industries, the free movement of labour and capital across international boundaries, the disappearance of ancient provincial centres under car parks and shopping malls and the globalisation of banking and finance were not simply economic variables but forces that radically transformed the

ways in which people thought and lived and even, to some degree, who they actually were.

(Harris, 2009: 16)

Such radical changes, wrought by globalization, might be expected to cause unease. But, as the 'Broken Britain' refrain suggests, even while living standards were rising and investment in public services increased (prior to the 2008 'crash') there was a popular sentiment that something was amiss, an 'ill-defined but widely pervasive sense of unease and social disintegration' (Harris, 2009: 6). To get a better grasp on these 'social evils' the Joseph Rowntree Foundation (JRF) ran a public consultation in 2007 which identified specific themes including individualism, consumerism and a decline of community, with tellingly, inequality and poverty (Utting, 2009).

What do you think? 4.1: The responsibility gap: transformation of communities?

Research for the Salvation Army (2004) identified similar themes to the JRF's 'social evils'. As well as rising individualism, consumerism and similar themes, the research identified three ways in which communities had been transformed:

1 **From communities of geography to communities of interest:** the argument here is that people increasingly 'define themselves according to their pastimes and interests rather than their birthplace, family network or cultural inheritance' (p. 42).
2 **From communities of necessity to communities of choice:** this involves a change 'from communities in which people associate with people, in places and under circumstances that they had not necessarily chosen, to those where they mix with people they have chosen, in locations they prefer and under circumstances which suit them' (p. 44).
3 **From permanent to transient communities:** whereas traditional communities were said to be permanent and involved people in long-term commitments, there has recently been 'an upsurge in "communities" which exist for only a brief period of time' (p. 44).

Questions for discussion

1 From your own experience and knowledge, do you agree that communities have changed in these ways?
2 If communities are being transformed in these ways, what do you think the implications are for social care?

Comment

The report acknowledges that the decline of community is often exaggerated but, nonetheless, holds that 'community spirit' as reflected in things like a sense of location, shared life experiences and interpersonal trust has declined. These and related changes, including the withdrawal of state welfare, are said to be creating 'a growing deficit of care for vulnerable groups' (Salvation Army, 2004: 7). One general practice implication is that social workers are more likely to work with service users and carers who are socially excluded in the sense of lacking informal support from family, friends and neighbours.

Social problems occur at all times of course, and to varying extents can be addressed by policy initiatives. However the JRF research used the term 'social evils' to emphasize that the issues are of a different nature: 'something more complex, menacing and indefinable and [which] may imply a degree of scepticism, realism or despair about whether any remedy can be found' (Harris, 2009: 5). In understanding why the problems are now more profound, two concepts are particularly relevant: neo-liberalism and, as indicated above, globalization. Globalization can be summarized as: 'the way that world trade, culture and technologies have become rapidly integrated . . . as geographic distance and cultural difference no longer pose an obstacle to trade' (War on Want, 2006: 9). Neo-liberalism is an ideology which since the 1980s has become almost synonymous with globalization. The essence of neo-liberalism is the promotion of free markets, privatization and the withdrawal of the state from public provision.

The globalization of the last 30 years has entailed an opening up of markets and increased trade internationally, the theory being that this increases economic growth. Yet Harvey (2005: 154) shows that, even before the 2008 downturn, 'neoliberalization has broadly failed to stimulate worldwide growth'. Although there was significant progress in reducing absolute poverty this was to a considerable extent due to spectacular economic growth in a few countries, particularly China and India. At the same time, a characteristic of neo-liberalism's 'distinctive form of globalization' (Harvey, 2005: 156) has been widening inequality. A 2005 review of the world social situation found that: 'economic and non-economic inequalities have actually increased in many parts of the world, and many forms of inequality have become more profound and complex in recent decades' (United Nations, 2005: 2). While the benefits of neo-liberal globalization are disputed, this finding does lend weight to Dominelli's (2010: 600) observation: 'that the heaviest price is exacted from poor people has become increasingly clear'.

In rich western countries these processes, Seabrook (2003: 9) argues, have rendered the poor invisible, having 'only walk-on parts in the great drama of progress' narrated by neo-liberalism. Seabrook uses the Victoria Climbié case to illustrate this invisibility; it is also an example of the growing impact of globalization on social work. In 1998 Victoria, then age 7, was taken from the Cote d'Ivoire to Paris by her great aunt, a French citizen, ostensibly to give her a chance of a better education. After her school raised a child at risk emergency notification about Victoria, her great aunt, Marie-Therese Kouao, brought her to London. Eight months later, in February 2000, Victoria, aged only 8, was dead, killed by the extreme abuse inflicted by Kouao and her partner Carl Manning. In moving in search of a better life from a relatively poor African country to one western metropolis and then another, all the time remaining hidden on the margins of society, Victoria followed a trail common to global population movements. That on her arrival in London Victoria remained a member of 'the invisible poor' stands as a warning to social workers. Despite Kouao and Manning having contact with many welfare agencies, in total 'encountering some 150 functionaries of the caring society', Victoria never attended school and 'was rarely spoken to by social workers'. The Climbié case is complex but despite the involvement of so many agencies and professionals 'Very little is known about the last four months of Victoria's life' (House of Commons Health Committee, 2003: 8). She was, Seabrook (2003: 18) concludes, 'virtually invisible'.

As much as it impacts on socially excluded people, social work has also not been spared the transformations wrought by neo-liberal globalization. Dustin (2007) summarizes these changes as the 'McDonaldization' of social work, meaning that the same principles on which McDonald's fast food outlets are run are increasingly being used to shape policy and practice in social work. McDonaldization is essentially a business model, a form of managerialism, in which 'services are regarded as commodities, objects or packages to be bought and sold' (2007: 31); much like burgers.

What do you think? 4.2: Globalization and social work practice

Listed below are some of the ways in which Dominelli (2010: 602) says social work practice has been affected by globalization.

- Disempowering social workers by restricting their access to resources that match their assessment of needs, particularly of those required by specific individuals.
- Shifting the practitioner–worker relationship away from relational social work to one that is more distant, as a result of the state's involvement in commissioning processes for services to be delivered by private and voluntary sector agencies.
- Reducing the impact of solidarity in service provision by moving away from universal services in favour of residual ones that target the neediest of the needy.
- Encouraging individual responsibility for meeting one's own needs while the state becomes preoccupied with competitiveness, opening the welfare market to international corporations keen to profit from their engagement in this field and supporting privatization.
- Increasing the impact of the international on local practice through the internationalization of social problems like poverty, the drug trade, trafficking in women and children . . .

Questions for discussion

1 Reflecting on your own knowledge and experience of social care, do you agree that social work is changing in the way Dominelli describes? Can you think of instances in practice which illustrate her points?
2 How do you think such changes might affect social work practice with poor and excluded people?

Comment

As society has changed so has social work, particularly since the introduction of care management in the 1990s. Dustin (2007) contrasts her 'Robin Hood' role, as a community social worker in the 1980s, when she used her professional discretion to help a poor family by giving them 'Section 1' money, with current performance-managed statutory social work. In the latter, she says, there is, 'dependence on technology in the form of computerized programmes to assess risk and the parallel loss of discretion associated with a deskilled social work role' (p. 7). This does not mean that social workers cannot alleviate service users' poverty and social exclusion but the opportunities to do so are more limited than they were, especially in statutory services. Partnership working, networking and advocacy are increasingly important for building alliances and accessing resources.

Social inequality: 'reading the riots'

Neo-liberal globalization has been a driving force of the changes which underlie concerns about 'Broken Britain'. If confirmation were needed that British society is broken, the rioting in English cities in August 2011 seemed to provide it. The unrest, looting and destruction was immense; in London alone the total cost including insurance claims and policing has been estimated at £30 million (Nwabuzo, 2012). The riots swept across England (although not to other parts of the UK): 'Images of people smashing shop windows, stealing, and setting fire to buildings were broadcast across the world' (Unwin in Low, 2011: 1). Amid the carnage that 'left people scratching their heads' searching for explanations, five people died.

For the government, explanations came on two levels. Prime Minister David Cameron lost no time in asserting that 'we know for sure . . . this was pure criminality' (quoted in Nwabuzo, 2012: 13). Official enquiries lent weight to this claim, finding that many rioters had criminal records. Yet the Riots, Communities and Victims Panel (2012) also identified wider factors, noting in particular an overlap between rioters and a group of some half a million 'forgotten families' who 'bump along the bottom of society'. The Panel did not use the term but these families are socially excluded. This is evident in the social character-istics of the rioters who were arrested and taken to court:

- they were young: about half (53 per cent) were aged 20 or younger;
- of those of school age, 42 per cent were receiving free school meals (the average for secondary schools is 16 per cent);
- nearly two thirds (64 per cent) lived in the 20 per cent most deprived areas in the country;
- and particularly in London and the West Midlands, they were disproportionately from Black ethnic groups (Nwabuzo, 2012).

Opportunistic looting, targeted at brands, was also identified as a feature of the riots. There is little doubt that this was linked to deprivation, research by the Children's Society showing that: '. . . many young people believe that poverty and disadvantage were one of the key reasons behind the August riots. We know from our work that there is a signifi-cant link between a child's material deprivation and their overall life satisfaction' (Chil-dren's Society, 2012).

The Panel's analysis supports this, showing that the 'brands' issue was linked to grow-ing inequality at a local level, with young, disadvantaged rioters feeling excluded from mainstream consumer culture. Surprisingly perhaps, Tim Morgan, global head of research at a financial markets company, wrote about the exclusionary effects of con-sumerism being urged on young people by 'big corporates and the media':

> 'You', young people are told, 'ought to live like this'. The second, flatly contradic-tory message is that 'you can't have it' . . . For a young person growing up in a non-rich household, the message, reinforced by peer pressure, is a deeply con-tradictory blend of 'this is fulfilment' and 'it will forever be out of your reach'.
> (Morgan, 2011: 2–3)

Ethnicity was also a factor in the riots; while there was a consensus that these were not 'race riots', research found that, especially for BME young men, police harassment through the use of stop and search, disadvantage and discrimination in education and employment all contributed to feelings of frustration and anger (Nwabuzo, 2012). All of these factors are linked to ideas about communities not working, as borne out by the JRF:

> Through our research, we know that people in some places feel absolutely pow-erless. And we know that many feel little loyalty to or involvement in their com-munities. We know that they believe their aspirations are frustrated and that whatever their effort they will not be recognised. People are worried about living

in a culture that has increasingly defined status through material possessions and the accumulation of possessions as worthy in its own right. We know about the devastating effects of recession on communities – with some never coming out of recession.

(Unwin in Low, 2011: 1)

The 2011 riots were symptomatic of the social changes which underlie the 'Broken Britain' and 'social evils' discourses, and to which poverty and social exclusion is integral. We should, however, be cautious of focusing exclusively on poverty and social exclusion without taking account of wider social relations, especially inequality. Relative poverty and social exclusion are concerned with people's ability to participate in normal social life and in this way they are linked to, although different from, inequality. Inequality is different because it looks at the whole society, not just those at the bottom. Dorling (2011) argues that the 2011 riots, like similar riots in the early 1980s, were linked to inequality. In both periods, rioting took place against a backdrop of recession, rising unemployment and cuts in services and benefits. Yet in the early 1980s Britain was a more equal society than it is now. From this, Dorling (2011) argues that it is not so much the extent of inequality that correlates with riots as its direction: growing inequality 'seeps through . . . into a collective, largely unconscious, well of despair' (p. 7).

Health inequalities and social work

Widening inequality may help to explain riots but there is also strong evidence that the scale of inequality is linked to, and probably causes, many other social problems. Not least of these are social inequalities in health: the fact that poor people suffer more illness and die younger than rich people. The extent of these inequalities can be shocking. The Marmot Review Team (2010) gives the example of a 17-year difference in average male life expectancy within a few miles in London: a wealthy part of Kensington and Chelsea where on average men live to age 88 compared to Tottenham Green where the average is only 71. In England as a whole the average difference in life expectancy between the poorest and the richest neighbourhoods is seven years. Moreover people in the richest areas enjoy 17 more years of disability-free life expectancy (Marmot Review Team 2010).

What do you think? 4.3: Why do poor people die young?

In 1980 *The Black Report* (Townsend and Davidson, 1982), the first government report on social inequalities in health, found wide class differences in both life expectancy and illness. Men and women in the 'unskilled manual' class, for example, were 2.5 times more likely to die before retirement age than those in the 'professional' class. The report reviewed four possible explanations of these inequalities:

1 **Artefact:** social class categories are artificial constructs which fail to adequately capture social reality. While statistics show that class differences in health persisted during the twentieth century, over the same period the manual working class became much smaller. Hence fewer people were in the groups with the worst health and to that extent health inequalities were diminishing.

2 **Natural or social selection:** healthier people will tend to move up the social scale (e.g. because their education and employment is not interrupted by illness) and people with poor health are likely to move in the opposite direction. Health inequalities may occur but they are natural or inevitable consequences of such trends.

3 **Cultural/behavioural:** a major cause of ill health, for poor people in particular, is their lifestyle; they are, for example, more likely to eat unhealthy diets and to smoke. The argument is that such behaviour is a matter of individual choice: people live like this because they choose to do so.

4 **Materialist or structuralist:** despite improved living standards in the twentieth century, socio-economic inequalities still render people in lower social classes vulnerable to poverty and other social disadvantages (e.g. bad housing, unsafe working conditions, etc.) which damage their health.

Questions for discussion

1 What do you think are the main strengths and weaknesses of each of the four explanations?
2 Of the four of them which one do you think offers the most convincing, or useful, explanation of health inequalities?

Comment

There is some substance to all four theories but the effects of the first three are relatively small; for instance, with the behavioural theory, most unhealthy behaviours are closely related to social status: poor, working-class people are less likely to have 'healthy lifestyles' than better-off people in higher social classes. This suggests that lifestyles are shaped more by social factors than by individual choice.

Understanding of the causes of health inequalities is much more sophisticated now than it was in the 1980s but a key finding of the *Black Report* still holds: 'that it is in some form or forms of the 'materialist' approach that the best answer lies' (Townsend and Davidson, 1982: 122). Put bluntly, poverty kills.

Social inequalities are evident in most measures of health and they usually occur as a social gradient: graduated inequalities between all groups in society getting worse the lower down the social scale you go. Figure 4.1 illustrates this with the example of smoking. The graph shows that people in the least affluent group smoke more than those in the next least affluent group who, in turn, smoke more than those in the next least affluent group to them and so on, up the scale. The graph also shows that as the overall prevalence of smoking declined between 1973 and 2004, the social gradient became steeper: that is, the poorer people were, the less likely they were to stop smoking. The reasons for this are discussed below but what both points show is that smoking, as with most risks to health, is closely related to social status and, especially, poverty.

Health inequalities are social in two ways. First, they are inequalities between groups in society whether defined by income, educational attainment, occupation or socio-economic status, gender or ethnicity. Second, the causes are primarily social rather than biological: health inequalities do not occur by chance and cannot be attributed simply to

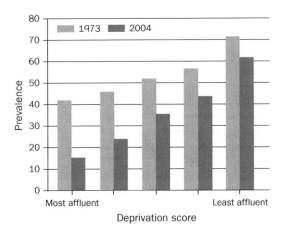

Figure 4.1 Cigarette smoking prevalence and deprivation in Great Britain, 1973 and 2004
Source: Department of Health (2008: 47)

genetics, 'bad' behaviour or restricted access to health care. Rather as the Marmot Review Team (2010: 37) says:

> Social inequalities in health arise because of inequalities in the conditions of daily life – the conditions in which people are born, grow, live, work and age – and the fundamental drivers that give rise to them: inequities in power, money and resources.

Educational attainment is closely related to health: people with more and higher qualifications are, in later life, likely to have higher incomes and better health and to live longer than people who 'fail' in school. Many factors influence children's chances in education and it is well established that the early years, particularly the first year of life, are crucial in the development of cognitive ability which, in turn, is a major determinant of life chances. As summarized by Marmot (2010: 63):

> ... birth weight, postnatal depression, being read to every day, and having a regular bed-time at age 3 are all likely to relate to a child's chances of doing well in school ... and [are] strongly influenced by parental income, education and socioeconomic status.

From the outset, parents' social status is a major factor in determining whether children are high or low achievers in school and,Marmot (2010: 63) adds, 'differences in early childhood tend to increase as children get older'. What happens in school is unlikely to overcome the social disadvantages of children's environment outside school.

Health inequalities and the 'inequities in power, money and resources' which cause them are structural, a product of unequal social relations. These are primarily class relations where social classes are based on exploitative economic relationships between groups in society: 'Stated simply, classes – like the working class, business owners, and their managerial class – exist in relationship to and co-define each other' (Krieger *et al.*, 1997, quoted in Rose and Hatzenbuehler, 2009: 462). Class and other systematic social inequalities, such as those of 'race' and gender, impact on health in complex ways, but fundamental to this is *embodiment*, meaning that the lived experience of poverty and inequality is, over lifetimes, incorporated physiologically: 'people's bodies (including their brains, minds and emotions) contain the cumulative impact of their material existence and its meaning, primarily as the outcome of unequal levels of stress and its biological impact' (Rose and Hatzenbuehler, 2009: 463). While class differences, arising from the fundamental relationships of capitalist society, might lie at the root of the most pervasive social inequalities in health, they are not the only cause. As Kreiger (1999: 265) says, 'Inequality hurts. Discrimination harms health.' The experience of being treated as a second class citizen whether by dint of class, gender, 'race' or disability, etc. will be embodied and will damage people's health – which is one reason why social inequalities in health are a social work issue.

When the issue is discussed in the media, health inequalities are usually presented as a lifestyle choice or a behavioural problem: poor people smoke, eat too much junk food and don't exercise. Whether stated explicitly or not, the message is all too often that it is a matter of individual choice. While there is some factual basis to this view (poor people are more likely to engage in most 'unhealthy behaviours') it is a superficial and inadequate explanation. It begs the question of why poor people behave in ways that will probably make them ill and eventually kill them. Health inequalities are better understood as a product of poverty and discrimination which is systemic and, Rose and Hatzenbuehler (2009) argue, inflicts psycho-social injuries on people. The experience of living on the wrong end of these inequalities will damage people's self-efficacy (a person's belief in their capacity to achieve) and self-esteem, which will likely give rise to heightened feelings of hopelessness and helplessness. As inequalities grow the extent of these injuries will probably grow too.

There are many reasons why poor people do things which in the long-term might damage their health. Often it is born of sheer practical necessity:

> If you live for more than six months on the minimum wage or on benefits there is growing evidence you cannot afford to buy the food you need for health. It is still to do with class but it's complex to unpick. Food is the flexible area that you cut back on when you are on a low income. Unlike council tax or utility bills, no one fines you if you don't spend on food and no one takes your children away, so that's what you cut, and you have a fag because that takes the hunger away.
> (Liz Dowler, professor of food and social policy,
> quoted in Lawrence, 2008)

These may be short-term coping strategies but people with few options tend to think in the 'here and now'. To look beyond that requires hope, and while social workers cannot 'change the world', they can work in partnership with service users to restore their self-efficacy, rebuild their self-esteem and thereby give them confidence that they can change their situation. Or, as Rose and Hatzenbuehler (2009: 467) put it, they can make poor people's 'struggles to live meaningful lives, a focal point for social work involvement'.

Doing this requires recognition that because health inequalities are primarily social in nature they are also preventable. Social conditions can be changed to alleviate what are called the social determinants of health inequalities. This is reflected in the growing recognition of health inequalities in social work. The International Federation of Social Work (2013: 7) states that 'All social workers should constantly question the health consequences of their actions'. Bywaters (2009) gives three reasons why health inequalities are a 'vital social work issue'. The first is to do with ethics and values: health inequalities are about human rights and social justice. Poor and excluded people not only die younger than others but the illness they experience is likely to bring pain and suffering which will blight their quality of life. This is unjust. Bywaters' second reason is that the determinants of health are primarily social and it is, at root, poverty and inequality that causes poor people to have worse health. The third reason is, in a sense, very practical. Poverty and poor health are two near-universal characteristics of the people social workers support: if they are not already suffering physical or mental ill-health, their probably impoverished living conditions are likely to put their health in jeopardy. Through their practice, social workers are very familiar with this but often fail to think about the health implications of clients' circumstances. To illustrate this, Bywaters (2009) gives the example of work with victims of domestic violence where social workers may be more preoccupied with the immediate presenting issues of safety, especially for any children involved, rather than thinking of the more long-term physical and mental health consequences for the women and their children.

What do you think? 4.4: Domestic violence, family poverty and children's health

This case study shows how underlying issues of poverty and social exclusion can damage children's physical and psychological health. It concerns a single-parent family, a mother with four children aged 14 (F), 9 (M), 7 (F) and 3 (F) years respectively, with multiple needs. The family were referred to the social worker by the primary school which the two middle children attended as they were being bullied because their uniforms were old and worn. The social worker was based in the school, working for a voluntary agency. Below, the social worker describes the family's situation and some of the steps she took to alleviate it.

> The children were very aware that they were poor and that there was no money for treats, for new school uniforms or for toys that were common among their peers. Mum was very intent on trying to take her family out of this impoverished position and was actually doing a combination of college and training. She didn't have money for formal childcare so various friends and neighbours looked after the children. The family had no relatives living nearby, but there was an aunt whom the family visited occasionally for 'weekends away'. In part, this isolation from family was as a result of the domestic violence – it's usually a feature for the perpetrator to cause a distance from support networks, not always geographical, but always emotional.
>
> The children found the variety of caregivers quite disconcerting, not because of concerns about their safety but just the chaos and absence of routine. It also created additional responsibilities for the 14-year-old, who often took the middle two to and from school. It changed the sibling relationships and the teen/Mum relationship: one minute the teen was a 'deputy parent' the next 'a child' . . .
>
> Mum also had to work shifts so again the children's lives were quite disrupted in terms of who was putting them to bed, who was having them at weekends, that kind of thing. There was also a sort of quid pro quo about childcare. This meant there was often another child in the household, sometimes overnight, and this child shared a bedroom with the three

youngest. The child was often unsettled at night, adding to sleeplessness. Meeting regularly with teachers was also important. They identified tiredness as an issue in class and [in terms of] the children's ability to fully access learning – this transpired to be caused by a combination of sleeplessness, child worries and hunger.

There was a history of domestic violence . . . and the children had witnessed some of it. It was ongoing, although the parents had separated and the violence was now sporadic, but it was significant in terms of emotional abuse of the children and contact was being dealt with in court. As with most perpetrators, contact was about meeting Dad's needs regardless of the impact on the children . . . The level of risk was such that the police were heavily involved as Dad had, for example, broken into the house and taken all the Christmas presents and thrown bricks through the windows . . . And because the children didn't have established relationships with some of their temporary caregivers, that added to their anxiety about whether they were safe from this man.

In terms of what you can do about it, listening to the children's worries, concerns and frustrations and then explaining to Mum how she could alleviate many of these stresses for her children. Using systemic family theory to understand how Mum's own experience of being parented was affecting her style of parenting helped her to see how crucial it is for parents to be consistent and to carry through with statements they make.

A combination of Mum being so focused on improving the financial future for her family and her own abusive childhood led to her not realizing the importance of experiences for the children in the present. For example, the children's fingernails were generally long and dirty and if fingernails were overlooked it is highly likely toenails were too – not having a routine often means things such as nail-cutting are over looked . . . These are not only visible signs of being unkempt, leading to taunts about hygiene, they can also lead to health problems.

Listening to Mum and appreciating how tired she was led to the development of a working relationship which provided opportunities to make suggestions about small, manageable change. For example, she used very simple things like a calendar with visual prompts to remind the children. When they forgot, because little children do, they could look at the calendar and there were little pictures and symbols which would tell them who was going to look after them and where they were going to be. Reward charts to target specific behaviours were also a useful way for Mum to ensure she paid attention to each child's needs and see improvements.

It could be said that the above is evidence of neglect. [Statutory] social care had been involved with the family when the physical violence was at a peak, but had closed the case once the physical threat to the children had 'been removed'.

I also talked to Mum about some preloved [second-hand] school uniforms which she accessed. She was also happy for me to talk to the school about the children attending a free breakfast club because part of the children's tiredness was the difficulty of finding the money for the right kind of food all the time.

So whilst I couldn't do anything about their finances, from the family feedback I was able to help Mum make a significant difference to the children: how they felt about themselves; how they felt about being at school; their physical growth and health and also their mental wellbeing.

Questions for discussion

1 Reflecting on the case study, what do you think might be the long-term consequences of the underlying poverty affecting this family?
2 Other than what the social worker has described, what other interventions might improve the life chances of this family?

Comment

If the children's situation was not improved, the conditions they were living in, for example, poverty, inconsistent care/neglect and witnessing domestic violence, would almost certainly have harmed their future development. This could have set them back in many areas of life including education, health and the ability to form stable relationships, all of which could lead to social exclusion in adult life.

The children's poor hygienic conditions and inadequate diet may have been affecting their health so the social worker may well have liaised with the health visitor or the GP about this. To tackle the family's social exclusion she might also have arranged access to any support groups provided by, for example, a local Sure Start children's centre. Another issue to address is income maximization; given the mother's hectic life (juggling work, study and parenting), benefit entitlement would be complex and families in situations like this often have debts. So accessing specialist advice, for example, from a Citizen's Advice Bureau, might have helped.

The life course

In seeing health inequalities from a social work perspective, the life course is a useful concept. Broadly this conceives of people's development over their lifespan as being continuous and cumulative, giving less emphasis to fixed life stages as compared, for example, to Erikson's eight stages of psycho-social development where the stages are quite rigid in terms of their age ranges and possible outcomes ('success' or 'failure'). Such theories can also be criticized as being ethno-centric, based on western life patterns, and ahistorical. Childhood, in particular, as a distinct phase of life, is largely a product of industrialization in western societies in the late nineteenth and twentieth centuries (Hunt, 2005). Early in the twenty-first century what people do at what point in their lives seems to be more fluid and varied. Bywaters (2007) contrasts, for example, the difference between care-leavers who are likely to have left education, set up home and have children before age 20, with the average (UK) age at which mothers have their first child, which was 29 in 2005. The latter is related to other changes: young people leaving the parental home later (in their mid-twenties); marrying later (or not at all) and higher rates of divorce and separation. The argument is not that stages in human development do not occur but rather that in a diverse and changing society they are varied and fluid, contingent upon the particular social context. The life course can be a more useful way of understanding human development because it is 'a dynamic concept which can be employed to explain how our lives flow through and around such stages' (Priestley, 2000: 424).

A useful approach to life course perspectives is to think in terms of a combination of two models.

1 **Critical period model:** where people make major transitions in their lives which can have long-term health and social effects. Such periods include starting, changing and leaving school, setting up home, becoming a parent and retirement. These periods are critical because they involve both material and psychological insecurity and uncertainty, which can have long-terms health impacts (Bartley et al., 1997).
2 **Accumulation of risk model:** this is that over their lifetime people are exposed to various factors which will influence their health for better or worse cumulatively throughout their life. A low birth-weight baby, born to an impoverished mother, is more likely as an adult to be in low-paid work with poor health and safety conditions and to enter retirement with little pension entitlement and poor health (Bywaters, 2007).

As a snapshot of how these two models can be combined, Bartley et al. (1997) cite research showing that children with slow growth up to age 7 were, when they were aged 22–32, three times more likely to be unemployed than children who had good growth. Height can serve as a proxy for social class (Dorling and Shaw, 2000) and while at an individual level these outcomes will be influenced by many variables, poverty and therefore diet will be a major influence on early growth. Disadvantage at this age has cumulative affects which might be decisive later when people enter the labour market, a critical period. What opportunities are open to people at that later point will of course greatly influence whether or not they are unemployed in their twenties.

Research on the long-term effects of psychological stress in childhood shows how a life course perspective can shed light on the interaction of biological, material and psycho-social influences over people's lives. To assess whether participants in the research had experienced childhood stress, they were asked if they had been separated from their mothers for more than one year. Those who had been separated were found to have high cortisol levels, cortisol being a hormone produced when people are stressed and which can be damaging to health. This matters to the life course because, 'early stress makes the child more susceptible to future stress, and this is reflected in patterns of higher cortisol levels' (Bartley, 2012: 16). As Bartley explains, people who suffer high stress in childhood are more likely to experience social and psychological problems in their adult lives:

> It is harder to concentrate in school, for example, so young people with stressful homes are less likely to get good qualifications and jobs. Emotional development may be adversely affected, leading to problems making adult relationships. Thus people who are more susceptible to stress also tend to accumulate less favourable experiences over a long period. This combination of stress-related risks may also lead people to develop more health-damaging behaviours, such as smoking, to help them cope.
>
> (Bartley, 2012: 17)

One of the advantages of a life course perspective, as this example shows, is that it can highlight patterns of how and when risks to health occur in people's lives. These can either be in chains, one risk leading to another, or in clusters, risks which are correlated but where the relationship is not necessarily causal; for example, a baby born into a poor family might have a low birth-weight and be exposed to passive smoking but one does not cause the other (Bywaters, 2007). In Bartley's (2012) research the link between childhood stress and poor health in later life was confirmed by looking at deaths five years after cortisol levels were measured: 'Patterns of cortisol that indicated higher levels of stress predicted increased death rates, particularly due to heart disease' (p. 17). There is, in other words, a direct relationship between psychological stress in childhood, biological change (high cortisol levels) and early death. And, as is discussed in Chapter 5, there is also a correlation between poverty and child maltreatment.

What do you think? 4.5: Social work and health inequalities

A life course perspective, then, both highlights the relevance of health inequalities to social work and can be helpful in translating this concern into practice. Bywaters (2007) draws out two important ways in which social workers can address health inequalities. First, as a life course perspective can bring out the cumulative impact of poverty and social exclusion on service users' lives, social workers should 'refocus attention on basic needs such as money, housing food and education, both in childhood and adult life' (2007: 143). Second, more emphasis should be given to history-taking in assessments; greater awareness of the biological, personal and social aspects of a service user's life course can increase insight into their current situation and their likely prospects. If risks, or 'insults' to health are then understood as occurring in chains and clusters, social workers can seek to alleviate risks and break causal chains through preventive work.

Questions for discussion

1 Do you agree with Bywaters' suggestions about how social workers can address health inequalities?
2 What policy changes might be necessary to help social workers more effectively tackle health inequalities?

Comment

How social work interventions can address health inequalities will vary according to the service user group and the nature of their needs and circumstances. However, while poverty causes ill health, the social determinants of health include all aspects of social life, so an eco-systems theory can be useful because this helps social workers take account of the full range of influences on service users' wellbeing.

Reducing health inequalities requires a preventive approach but, as is discussed in Chapter 5 in relation to children's services, while social policy has of late shifted more towards prevention, social work has often been marginal to this. Social workers in the voluntary sector usually have more scope for preventive work but statutory social work should be given a much more central role in prevention, not least because social work skills and knowledge are well-suited for this role.

Poverty, parenting and teenage pregnancy

A theme of the 'Broken Britain' discourse is family breakdown and the decline in marriage. The coalition government's *Social Justice* White Paper points out that 'Marriage rates have more than halved in the last 40 years, while the number of lone parent households increased by an average of 26,000 a year from the early 1980s to 2010' (Secretary of State for Work and Pensions, 2012: 6). This is presented as part of 'The Scale of the Challenge' in the government's strategy of 'tackling poverty in all its forms' (p. 4). The proposed response to this challenge strongly endorses marriage: 'Government believes marriage often provides an excellent environment in which to bring up children. So the Government is clear that marriage should be supported and encouraged' (p. 16).

Marriage, or rather the absence of it, family breakdown and poverty have long been intertwined in debates about the causes and consequences of poverty and exclusion. From the 1990s to the early 2000s the main concern was about single parents, especially teenage parents. This is a heavily gendered way of looking at social disadvantage: most teenage parents are unmarried and most single parents are women (SEU, 1999). It is linked to what has been called 'the feminization of poverty'. This is the relatively recent recognition of an old problem: that women are at greater risk of poverty than men, are more likely to experience recurrent and longer spells of poverty and the effects of childhood poverty are likely to be greater on them. The increase in female-headed households, particularly single mothers, has made this situation more visible (Lister, 2004).

Discussion of single parents becomes explicitly gendered when mothers are presented as being a cause of their families' poverty. In the 1990s, the Conservative government portrayed lone mothers as 'a threat to the fabric of society . . . rearing delinquent children while scrounging benefits' and jumping the queue for council housing (Duncan *et al.*, 1999: 238). Subsequently, teenage pregnancy became a priority in the Labour government's drive to reduce social exclusion from 1997. Labour's response to the moral panic about teenage pregnancy illustrates two aspects of poverty and social exclusion which were outlined in Chapter 2. The first is the 'othering' and stigmatization of, in this case, young women. The second is human agency – that people in poverty and social exclusion are not passive victims but can and do act to change their situation.

Labour's Teenage Pregnancy Strategy was a 10-year preventative programme with targets, to:

1 Reduce the rate of teenage conceptions with the specific aim of halving the rate of conceptions among under-18s, and to set a firmly established downward trend in the rate of conceptions among under-16s, by 2010 [and]
2 Increase the participation of teenage parents in education, training and employment to 60% by 2010, to reduce their risk of long-term social exclusion.
(Dennison, 2004: 1)

The SEU (1999) report which informed the Strategy painted an alarming picture, reflecting the view that teenage pregnancy was a factor in a wider social crisis. After pointing out that teenage birth rates were much higher here than in other western European countries, the report claimed that, for example,

The facts are stark: this is a problem which affects just about every part of the country ... But it is far worse in the poorest areas and among the most vulnerable young people, including those in care and those who have been excluded from school.

(SEU, 1999: 6)

The SEU also argued that teenage pregnancy was a risk factor for many forms of poverty and exclusion. It was acknowledged that the causes were complex but three key factors were singled out:

- Young people's **low expectations**: the report claimed that a cause of the UK's high rates of teenage pregnancy was that 'there are more young people who see no prospect of a job and fear they will end up on benefit one way or the other. Put simply, they see no reason not to get pregnant' (SEU, 1999: 7).
- Their **ignorance**: young people, it was said 'do not know how easy it is to get pregnant and how hard it is to be a parent' (SEU, 1999: 7).
- **Mixed messages**: young people were bombarded with messages apparently promoting sexual activity while discussion of contraception and safe sex was swept under the carpet.

Despite the conclusion that these problems resulted from society's neglect, presenting the issues in these terms risked pathologizing young parents, 'low expectations and ignorance' is not that far removed from fecklessness.

Labour's strategy did provide valuable support to pregnant young women and mothers; nonetheless Arai (2009: 172) argues that in associating teenage pregnancy so strongly with social exclusion it 'had a major negative consequence'. Rather than challenging negative stereotypes it reinforced the view of teenage mothers as a social problem. The effect, Arai suggests, was to present them as a 'demographic residuum', suffering 'fertility induced social exclusion' which isolated them from a society modernizing under the impact of globalization:

The young mother – welfare dependent, geographically immobile, poorly educated and with apparently limited vision – is the antithesis of this agenda. In modern, advanced, highly skilled and fast-changing industrial societies, the worst thing to be is a residuum of any kind. In this kind of economic setting, early parenthood is represented as an archaic and chronically self-limiting behaviour.

(Arai 2009: 181)

As the majority of teenage pregnancies are unplanned (SEU, 1999), human agency is exercised when the decision is made whether to have the baby or not. Young women whose aspirations are apparently in tune with the times are, it seems, 'clear and decisive in their choice of abortion' (Lee *et al.*, 2004: 48). These are women who have their sights set on higher education and a career after that. But for many women who choose not to terminate their pregnancies the decision need not be negative either in intent or outcome:

On the contrary, it can appear to provide direction in life, the opportunity to take personal responsibility and, in some cases, a close personal relationship with a valued other. Some young women from deprived backgrounds therefore find the prospect of motherhood attractive.

(Lee *et al.*, 2004: 48)

Arai also found that early motherhood can be positive:

> For those young women who had previously had fraught relationships with parents, birth transformed family dynamics and healed breaches. For young women who had experienced the worst kinds of adversity, birth was described as a direct response to this ... In families and social networks where early fertility is relatively common, young women are likely to be accepted and well supported.
>
> (Arai, 2009: 175, 180)

For young working class women living in deprived areas the decision to have a baby, even if made after conception, can be a rational response to the realities of their social situation. In this context a policy agenda which exhorts socially excluded young women to delay childbirth is alien, showing little appreciation of the realities of their lives. From a social work perspective this is disempowering, because it denies the validity of teenage parents' agency in deciding to have children.

What do you think? 4.6: Young women, social exclusion and group work

In the case study below, social workers in a family centre begin by discussing how poverty can lead to social exclusion for service users; who are mainly young women, many of them single parents and often child protection cases. The social workers then describe how group work can be used, with one-to-one work, to overcome isolation and promote inclusion.

> Very few of our clients *ever* go away [on holiday]. Lots of kids who come here have never been to the seaside, and we're not far away. Their lives are lived within a certain area and that's it. That must be linked to money and lack of expectation.
>
> I think that's the saddest part about poverty: you lose any aspirations . . . I don't think any of our clients, or very few, would ever think to discuss going to uni, or travelling the world, or doing a gap year . . . And because they don't think about it for themselves, they wouldn't think about it for their children.
>
> We run a teenage girls group for children who are looked-after or are on the edge of care, are child protection cases. They haven't got much of a sense of identity, have had real issues at home. They've got so many problems they wouldn't rock up to a normal youth club or anything like that, they just wouldn't fit in. But they do here, they are a very inclusive group. They will access the community; they will, for example, go to carol services at Christmas and to activity days. Most of them have never done that kind of thing.
>
> Groups in themselves can be very empowering: the fact that they are coming together and have got a shared experience, often they will make friends within the groups. We've got one at the moment that is really gelling: they're getting that kind of support within the group and they are meeting and travelling here together, they've exchanged phone numbers

and they're meeting outside the group. So the group, by default, helps with social exclusion.

Part of the work is 'practical', signposting to other services or flagging up things frontline teams might be able to help with, with their Section 17 money . . . And more broadly part of it would be self-esteem work, solution focused therapy and goal setting. If we've got a family where the mother wants to go to college we might look at that as part of direct work . . .

Questions for discussion

1 How far do you think the intervention the social workers describe can overcome social exclusion and poverty?
2 In social policy terms what else is needed to make the work carried out by the family centre team more sustainable?

Comment

When they were interviewed the social workers were particularly enthusiastic about how group work could empower service users and help them change their lives. This does suggest that, with the support of other agencies, they can significantly reduce social exclusion and poverty and build service users' resilience and support networks. What the social workers probably cannot do is transform the services users' material circumstances. Income maximization, for instance, can ease families' budgeting problems but is unlikely to lift them far above the poverty line.

In policy terms, given that many of the families live in 'hard-to-let' social housing, more and better affordable housing would probably help, particularly, for instance, for mothers fleeing domestic violence. As is alluded to by the social workers, if benefit rules were relaxed to encourage young mothers to return to education that would probably make changing their situation seem more realistic and sustainable to the service users.

More recently, especially under the coalition government from 2010, the policy focus has been less on lone mothers specifically and more on parenting and poverty generally (Dermott, 2012). Or rather, the government seems to want to improve children's development while downplaying poverty as a causal factor in this. Greeting a research report on poor parenting, David Cameron claimed, in January 2010, that: 'the differences in child outcomes between a child born in poverty and a child born in wealth are no longer statistically significant when both have been raised by "confident and able parents"' (quoted in Sparrow, 2010). Cameron could hardly contain his enthusiasm for the research results:

It would be over the top to say that it is to social science what E = MC2 was to physics, but I think it is a real "sit up and think" moment. That discovery defined the laws of relativity; this one is the new law for social mobility . . . What matters most to a child's life chances is not the wealth of their upbringing but the warmth of their parenting.

(quoted in Sparrow, 2010)

Cameron did acknowledge that it was easier to be a 'warm' parent if you were wealthy, but part of his agenda was to minimize the significance of cash benefits when his government was making major cuts in the welfare budget. Labour MP Frank Field's (2010) 'independent review on poverty and life chances' published later that year was complementary to this agenda. The review sought to provide an alternative strategy to what Field called Labour's 'income transfer approach' to reducing child poverty (i.e. using the tax and benefits system to increase the incomes of families in poverty). While acknowledging that 'good services matter too', Field (p. 7) argued:

> The things that matter most are a healthy pregnancy; good maternal mental health; secure bonding with the child; love and responsiveness of parents along with clear boundaries, as well as opportunities for a child's cognitive, language and social and emotional development.

He also claimed that, 'It is family background, parental education, good parenting and the opportunities for learning and development in those crucial years that together matter more to children than money' (p. 7).

What do you think? 4.7: Parenting and poverty

Questions for discussion

1 How do you think parenting relates to poverty and social exclusion? Why do you think there has been a change in social policy (discussed above) with more emphasis being given to parenting and less to poverty as influences on children's wellbeing?

Comment

Although the coalition government does not explicitly recognize social exclusion, in terms of Levitas' three discourses (discussed in Chapter 3) its policy pronouncements about 'scroungers' and 'welfare' dependency, etc., are very much part of a MUD (moral underclass) discourse. This fits with their wider policy agenda in two ways:

1 It puts primary responsibility for their situation on poor/excluded people themselves. In this case the difficulties children in poor families have are portrayed as being mainly caused by their parents' inadequacies rather than the fact that they are usually living on very low incomes.
2 If this is the case, it legitimizes the cuts in benefits which the government has introduced, which is in accord with its general austerity programme of cutting public spending.

Adopting this MUD discourse pathologizes and stigmatizes parents who are struggling with poverty.

To a large extent, Field's argument contrasting parenting with income is a false dichotomy. Certainly no social worker would argue that the warm, nurturing parenting Field describes is unimportant to child development. However, what is missing from this discourse about poverty and parenting is due recognition of the importance of money.

To paraphrase Strelitz and Lister (2008: 144): 'at the centre of the experience of poverty is lack of income'. Money matters in different ways. In education what Field calls 'family background' can have indirect effects: parents in low-income families are likely to be younger than average, less well educated and have more children; all factors likely to militate against their children's educational achievement (Gregg, 2008). Then there are the direct effects of low income: typically poor parents struggling to pay for school uniforms and trips. Overall, Gregg estimates that about 50 per cent of educational inequality, 'the gaps in attainment between rich and poor, stem from differences in income' (Gregg, 2008: 78). While Field's recommendations for high-quality support for parents and children were welcomed by child poverty experts there was also criticism of his suggestion that this should come at the expense of the incomes of poor families (Barnardo's, 2011; Child Poverty Action Group 2011). Even if Field's argument was sound, with deep spending cuts on children's social care, particularly in preventive services and in both statutory and voluntary sectors, the prospects for high-quality children's services are not rosy (Chartered Institute of Public Finance and Accountancy 2011; Action for Children, 2012).

While the coalition government acknowledges that poverty and poor parenting are linked, there is simultaneously a denial of the significance of poverty as a cause of social problems. As Dermott (2012) points out, this paradoxical position was articulated in David Cameron's condemnation of the 2011 riots, particularly in his assertions that 'these riots were not about poverty' but were about behaviour for which parents were culpable: 'Well, join the dots and you have a clear idea about why some of these young people were behaving so terribly. Either there was no one at home, they didn't much care or they'd lost control' (Cameron quoted Dermot, 2012: 2).

If, for the rioters there were 'no parents at home' as they grew up, given that they were mainly from deprived areas it might be helpful to consider why that was. In discussing why children from poor families are more likely to display aggressive behaviour as adults, Marmot (2004) cites an analogy with gardening to contrast differences between rich and poor. To see, he says, 'the grossest effects of maternal deprivation visit your local prison' (p. 236). His point is that prison populations are largely made up of men and, increasingly, women who are likely to have, variously, been looked-after children, have poor literacy and/or mental health problems. In the relationship between poverty, parenting and children's outcomes there is a double bind. Poverty impacts on parenting: it is harder to be a good parent if you are poor. But for poor families, parental 'tending' is more important in helping children overcome the disadvantages of growing up in an impoverished, 'less fertile' environment: 'The differences among flowers that are growing in fertile ground will be mainly due to [inherited] genotype differences, whereas differences among flowers growing in less fertile ground will be due to the quality of the added care (for example, water, fertilizer) given' (Tremblay quoted in Marmot, 2004: 237). Here too there is a social gradient: the higher the socio-economic position the less the family, or parenting, matter to the prevalence of aggressive behaviour, because the children are growing up in 'fertile ground'. At the bottom of the social scale, family has more significance for outcomes, positive or negative. In this stony ground more water and fertilizer is needed but, being poor, it is harder to provide (for reasons discussed in Chapter 5).

In 2007 UNICEF published a 'Report Card' on child wellbeing in 21 rich countries in Europe and North America. Countries were ranked according to how their children fared under six different headings:

- material wellbeing;
- health and safety;
- education;

- peer and family relationships;
- behaviours and risks;
- young people's own subjective sense of wellbeing.

Overall, the UK, one of the richer of these rich countries, came bottom. Of the six measures the UK was last or second last on three: peer and family relationships, behaviours and risks, and subjective wellbeing. All three are linked to the arguments about parenting discussed above. In his book *Status Syndrome*, Michel Marmot (2004) argues that social status is a major determinant of health in wealthy countries. To show this he gives the example of Hollywood movie stars among whom Oscar winners live on average four years longer than their co-stars and other actors who were nominated for but did not win Oscars. Film stars are by definition privileged – the point here is that the *extra* status afforded by having an Oscar makes a difference even among this elite group, a difference equivalent to 'reducing your chances of dying from a heart attack to zero' (Marmot, 2004: 22). Marmot's general argument is that social status is a major determinant of health because it shapes autonomy and social participation: 'the lower in the [social] hierarchy you are, the less likely it is that you will have full control over your life and opportunities for full social participation' (p. 248). Working with service users to promote social participation, develop their autonomy and enhance their self-respect is very much the 'core business' of social work.

An argument very similar to Marmot's has been advanced to explain the prevalence of a much wider range of social problems, beyond health inequalities. In *The Spirit Level*, Richard Wilkinson and Kate Pickett (2009) argue that income inequality is an underlying cause of many social problems in rich developed countries. They do this by showing a correlation between the extent of income inequality and 38 social issues or problems: the greater the income inequality there is in a society the more common a social problem will be. Wilkinson and Pickett's analysis has developed from research into the causes of health inequalities and, accordingly, emphasizes social gradients and the significance of status. In the UK there is, for example, a social gradient in teenage pregnancy: 'Each year almost 5 per cent of teenagers in the poorest quarter of homes have a first baby, four times the rate in the richest quarter. But even in the second richest quarter . . . the rate is double that of the richest . . .' (p. 121).

Teenage pregnancy does most affect the poor but it also affects all groups higher up the social scale, in inverse relation to their social status. It is also more common in more unequal societies. The USA, the most unequal country discussed in *The Spirit Level*, has a teenage birth rate over four times the EU average and more than 10 times higher than the rate in Japan, the least unequal country in the study. Beneath these broad figures lie significant differences related to the cultures of particular societies. In some countries teenage mothers are much more likely to be married; Japan not only has fewer teenage mothers but 86 per cent of them are married, compared to less than 25 per cent in the USA, UK and New Zealand. In these more unequal societies, high rates of teenage pregnancy are also, Wilkinson and Pickett (2009: 124) say, 'associated with the broad range of health and social problems that we think of as typical consequences of early motherhood'. There are also variations within societies – for example, some ethnic minority groups which have high rates of poverty and exclusion (see Chapter 3) also have above average rates of teenage pregnancy but most Bangladeshi teenage mothers are likely to be married (SEU, 1999). So while the general relationship between income inequality and social problems is particularly relevant to the UK, because it is a very unequal society, at the level of practice we should still be sensitive to cultural variations.

The Spirit Level has attracted a lot of publicity, probably because it is in tune with the zeitgeist, the mood of the times. It can for instance be seen as offering an explanation for the 'social evils' discussed earlier. The book addresses issues which go to the heart of 'how we live now', asking inherently political questions about the distribution of resources and life chances in society. Probably because of this, *The Spirit Level* has been much criticized. However, an independent review concluded that its methods are robust and that its central argument about the correlation between income inequality and health and social problems is good (Rowlingson, 2011). Correlation is not cause, nonetheless *The Spirit Level* makes a compelling case that the extent of income inequality, used as a proxy for wider social inequality and stratification, does have a causal effect on many social problems. As Wilkinson and Pickett argue, the fact that all the social problems which increase with inequality also show a strong class gradient (i.e. they are more common in more unequal societies and more common the further down the social scale you go within societies) does suggest the relationship is causal.

One clear message of *The Spirit Level* is that economic growth will not by itself improve wellbeing in society or, to put it another way, will not mend 'Broken Britain'. If the 'social evils' are to be expunged, or at least ameliorated, it follows that we should instead prioritize the quality of social relations by, in particular, reducing social inequalities. Creating a more equal society might seem far removed from the day-to-day realities of social work practice but the quality of social relations is very much a social work concern, as are service users' autonomy and social participation. *The Spirit Level* and an understanding of the social determinants of health can inform social work practice in at least three ways.

First, it provides compelling evidence of the harmful effects of neo-liberal policies. Despite a probably temporary fall in 2010–11, income inequality is as high now as it was when New Labour won the 1997 general election (Cribb *et al.*, 2012). With 'austerity' and welfare reform, the likelihood is that social inequalities will get worse before they get better. *The Spirit Level* provides social workers with a critique of the social impact of these policies. The four countries with the least unequal income distribution, Japan, Norway, Sweden and Finland, are also those which have the lowest prevalence of social problems. None of them are utopias, nor are they unaffected by neo-liberal globalization, but they do show that is it possible to do things differently. The argument that 'there is no alternative' is false.

Second, *The Spirit Level* can help social workers contextualize service users' lives and the issues confronting them. Teenage pregnancy, failing in school, mental distress, imprisonment and drug use all increase when inequality grows. And child wellbeing falls. These facts encapsulate a powerful argument against pathologizing service users. The families and individuals social workers support vary, all have their own traits and circumstances, but they are also powerfully affected by the social environment in which they live. Yet, as we have seen with teenage mothers, while their responses to those structural constraints might be at odds with what their 'betters' prescribe, it is often a rational attempt to make the best of being trapped in poverty and social exclusion by forces beyond their control.

Third, as we have seen, *The Spirit Level* and *Status Syndrome* are concerned with the psycho-social impact of inequality on people's lives and how we respond to their analysis will depend on our ethics and values. Having low status in hierarchical societies exacerbates the depredations of material hardship because we are social beings:

> For a species which thrives on friendship and enjoys cooperation and trust, which has a strong sense of fairness . . . it is clear that social structures which create relationships based on inequality, inferiority and social exclusion must inflict a great deal of social pain.
>
> (Wilkinson and Pickett, 2009: 213)

Marmot (2004: 254) argues that we should care about health inequalities 'where they are the result of unfairness that could be put right'. One implication of the social gradient is that if some groups in society can enjoy better health and wellbeing there is at least the potential for poor people to do the same. This is a matter of social justice, which is integral to social work and which runs counter to the flow of neo-liberal globalization. These are difficult times but, whatever the obstacles, social workers do generally have more autonomy and status than their clients. They also have a professional obligation to use such resources to counter poverty and social inequality. Or, as Craig (2002: 679) puts it, 'social workers can play an important role as facilitators and advocates for those most on the margins of society, and [can help] to "make the invisible visible"'.

Summary of main points

- Since the 1980s the UK has undergone profound socio-economic changes, giving rise to concerns about a deep social crisis characterized by individualism, consumerism and high levels of poverty and social exclusion.
- These developments are linked to neo-liberal globalization which has impacted on social work through what Dustin (2007) calls the 'McDonaldization of social work': the adoption of business methods and ideology in social work policy and practice.
- Social inequalities in health are a consequence of the psycho-social impact of living in very unequal societies, caused by poor and excluded people being denied control over their lives and social participation.
- As health inequalities are socially determined and linked to lack of autonomy and social participation, social workers are well placed to address them.
- High social inequality increases the prevalence of many of the social problems social workers encounter in practice.
- Social work's ethical commitment to social justice and empowerment obliges practitioners to work with service users to alleviate the health and other consequences of such inequality.

Further reading by topic

Globalization and neo-liberalism

Dominelli, L. (2010) Globalization, Contemporary Challenges and Social Work Practice, *International Social Work*, 53.5, 599–612.

Harvey, D. (2005) *A Brief History of Neoliberalism*, Oxford: Oxford University Press.

Health inequalities

Bywaters, P., McLeod, E. and Napier, L. (eds) (2009) *Social Work and Global Health Inequalities: practice and policy developments*, Bristol: Policy Press.

Marmot, M. (2004) *Status Syndrome: how your social standing directly affects your health and life expectancy*, London: Bloomsbury.

Social inequality

Wilkinson, R. and Pickett, K. (2009) *The Spirit Level: why more equal societies almost always do better*, London: Allen Lane.

Useful websites

Social Work and Health Inequalities Network: www2.warwick.ac.uk/fac/cross_fac/healthatwarwick/research/devgroups/socialwork/swhin

The Equality Trust (is linked to, and has resources related to *The Spirit Level*): www.equalitytrust.org.uk

5 Children and families: poverty, abuse and practice

Key messages

- Poverty and social exclusion can cause child abuse at family, community and societal levels.
- The 'artificial divide' in policy and practice between prevention and protection inhibits social workers' capacity to tackle families' poverty and social exclusion.
- An ecological perspective should underpin practice with children and families because it highlights the ways poverty can damage families and informs holistic responses to that poverty.

> Poor children are deprived of material assets, they experience higher mortality and morbidity, their activities and opportunities are constrained, they are more likely to suffer mental ill-health and they are more likely to live in poor housing and poor neighbourhoods . . . Child poverty is thus a very powerful indicator of the well-being of children.
>
> (Bradshaw, 2011b: 28)

Bradshaw's summary of the ways children's lives are blighted by poverty will be familiar to social workers working with children and families. This chapter examines how social workers can work with families to alleviate these effects. We look first at the relationship between poverty and child abuse, particularly neglect. This is then related to the tension in policy and practice between prevention and early intervention on the one hand and child protection on the other. The argument is that social workers can most effectively tackle child poverty by taking an ecological perspective which locates family poverty and exclusion in its social context. Among the advantages of an ecological approach are that it encourages working in partnership with families, understanding their perspective on problems and utilizing their strengths in tackling them, and it facilitates a community orientation to practice.

Poverty and child abuse

As we saw in Chapter 2, although the number of children in poverty fell under the Labour government to 2010, that downward trend is now being reversed. For the foreseeable future the context of social work with children and families is going to be one of high and rising levels of poverty which will bring growing need:

> By 2015 there will be significantly more children living within vulnerable families than there were in 2008; they will be significantly worse off in terms of disposable income; and . . . the public spending cuts [in services] will have also hit them hard.
>
> (Reed, 2012: 9)

Child abuse, especially neglect, the most common form of abuse (Rose, 2010), could be added to Bradshaw's summary of the effects of the poverty (above). An early national study of child maltreatment found that victims of abuse and neglect were twice as likely as the average to have grown up in families where money was short (Cawson, 2002). A more recent report confirmed that higher rates of maltreatment among disadvantaged families have persisted (Radford *et al.*, 2011). The forms of maltreatment most associated with poverty and social exclusion are neglect and, to a lesser extent, physical abuse; sexual and emotional abuse are less clearly linked to socio-economic conditions (for a review see Dyson, 2008). There is though a class bias in that the association between poverty and some forms of abuse is related to the fact that poor working-class families are subjected to greater surveillance than middle-class families. Moreover 'respectable' professional families are also treated differently than poor people. These points are manifestations of the fact that child abuse is a social construct: what it is thought to be, who is affected (victims and perpetrators) and how it is dealt with are shaped by the social context and thus by social divisions of class, gender and 'race', etc. (Hooper, 2011; Rogowski, 2013).

In relation to gender, for example, women, particularly ethnic minority women, are not only more likely to be poor than men, they are also more prone to recurrent poverty and to being poor for longer periods. This has consequences for child wellbeing because as mothers 'Women are also the main managers of family poverty' (Women's Budget Group, 2005: iii). Inevitably this takes a toll on women's physical and mental health, particularly where they are in debt and/or victims of domestic violence. Associated feelings of guilt and shame, lack of control and depression can also lead to social exclusion, as can having to relocate to escape domestic violence with the risk of losing sources of social support. So while domestic violence occurs in all classes, it is associated with poverty and exclusion (Hooper *et al.*, 2007) and 'the causes and consequences of poverty are intertwined in a vicious circle' (Women's Budget Group, 2005: iii). Witnessing domestic violence, a form of emotional abuse, can be among the consequences for children.

As was discussed in Chapter 3, ethnic minorities are twice as likely to be poor as the White British majority and over half of Bangladeshi and Pakistani children grow up in poverty (Platt, 2009). Despite the greater need resulting from such poverty and isolation, Owen and Statham (2009: 13) found that 'minority ethnic families are less well served by family support services'. In general, the relationship between need and support received from children's services is characterized by 'disproportionality': 'on average, children of mixed ethnic groups and Black children are over-represented in the child welfare statistics and Asian children are under-represented' (Owen and Statham, 2009: 2–3). The causes of this are not fully understood but there is some evidence that ethnic minority children's needs are recognized late, at crisis point, and hence as child protection cases (Owen and Statham, 2009) rather than being addressed earlier by preventive services. Victoria Climbié's 'invisibility' to children's services (see Chapter 4) is a particularly tragic example of this. Indeed, Garrett (2009) argues that the significance of 'race' was 'partitioned off' and possibly downgraded in the Laming Inquiry into Victoria's death and in the subsequent *Every Child Matters* agenda, while Chand (2008) seems to suggest that racism should be recognized as a form of child abuse.

As much as child maltreatment is affected by gender and 'race' so too it is shaped by poverty and social exclusion. However, an essential caution here is that 'the majority of families living in extremely disadvantaged circumstances do manage to provide safe, nurturing and loving environments for children' (Spencer and Baldwin, 2005: 31). That said, one way to begin to unpick the relationship between poverty and abuse is to examine the problem at three overlapping levels: family, community and society.

The statutory guidance for safeguarding children defines neglect as: 'The persistent failure to meet a child's basic physical and/or psychological needs, likely to result in the serious impairment of the child's health or development . . . [including failure to] provide adequate food, clothing and shelter' (HM Government, 2013: 86). For families in poverty, neglect in this material sense can be a constant threat. In their research with poor families, Hooper *et al.* (2007: 18) found that 'over a quarter could not afford a cooked main meal each day for each adult, and nearly half could not afford basic toys and sports gear for children or a day trip once a year'. Impoverished mothers going without meals and making other sacrifices for their children is common but children are also often sensitive to their parents' difficulties and try to alleviate them by hiding their own needs. Hooper *et al.* also found that 14 per cent of parents could not afford a cooked meal every day for their children and nearly one third could not afford warm winter clothing for them either. As evidence of material neglect this raises questions of responsibility which go beyond individual families: does society not have a responsibility to provide poor families with enough money to feed their children?

What do you think? 5.1: Living with hardship: going without

Figure 5.1 is taken from the *Living with Hardship* (Hooper *et al.*, 2007) report on families in poverty and shows the proportion of parents who said they could not afford various items. The items listed are similar to those used in the 'Breadline Britain' surveys (1983–2012) discussed in Chapter 2.

Questions for discussion

1 Which of the items listed in the graph do you think are necessities; that is, in your opinion what things do people need to be able to participate in 'normal social life'?
2 Does seeing the proportion of families that do not have particular items change what you think are necessities – for example, does the fact that nearly half of the families cannot afford a day trip once a year suggest that this should not be seen as a necessity?

Comment

Comparing Hooper *et al.*'s findings with the 'Breadline Britain' surveys does indicate how excluded families can be. For example, there are two items which have

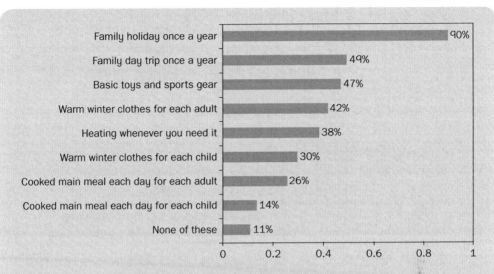

Figure 5.1 Proportion (%) of parents in poor families who could not afford selected items

Source: Hooper et al. (2007: 18)

consistently had very large majority support (c. 80–90 per cent) as necessities, yet significant proportions of these poor families cannot afford:

- warm clothing for either adults and/or children;
- being able to adequately heat their homes.

Given that the families in the *Living with Hardship* study are likely to have had contact with social services, this does perhaps emphasize just how poor such families often are.

Looking beyond material factors, parental stress is the most widely cited causal factor in the relationship between poverty and neglect (Dyson, 2008). Stress can come from many sources; living with little money brings uncertainty because of fluctuations in income (e.g. when benefit entitlement changes) and outgoings (e.g. when fuel bills rise or appliances break down). Trying to 'make ends meet' without an adequate income is time consuming because it requires planning and careful shopping, often 'robbing Peter to pay Paul'. Poverty also takes a psychological toll because, when even basic items become luxuries, the difficulty of affording them reminds mothers that they 'ain't got what everyone else has got' (Hooper *et al.*, 2007: 19).

The *Living with Hardship* research is particularly useful because many of the participants were recruited via children's services so their experiences are probably much like those of the families social workers support in practice. As well as low income, bad housing and other material factors, most of the parents were struggling with other problems, 'including histories of ongoing abuse (rape by boyfriends and others as well as childhood maltreatment and domestic violence) mental and physical ill-health, relationship breakdown and bereavement' (Hooper *et al.*, 2007: 43). The prevalence of these problems among the parents is a sharp manifestation of social inequalities in health, as discussed in Chapter 2. Their lives show starkly how lack of status and autonomy generates psycho-social stress and undermines health. Compounded by poverty, the problems these parents have to cope with often left them 'struggling to exercise control and authority over their lives' (2007: 43).

That living like this is stressful hardly needs saying; that it can lead to neglect by sapping parents' energy for nurturing activities with their children (Hooper *et al.*, 2007) also seems apparent. Single-parent families, usually lone mothers, are likely to be worst affected both because they are more likely to be poor and because of time constraints and related issues: generally it will be harder for one parent to give children the attention that two parents can. That children in single-parent households are less likely to eat or talk with their parents and are more likely to engage in risky behaviour (Tomlinson and Walker, 2009) might then be expected.

The psycho-social impact of poverty on parenting, which can lead to neglect, has a community, or local, aspect which, in turn, has several dimensions which vary according to the particular context. Living in the circumstances described above is not likely to boost parents' self-esteem, particularly given the stigma that is attached to poor people, especially if they are reliant on welfare benefits. One effect of low self-esteem and stigma can be to isolate poor families.

The social support available to parents is a key factor in helping them have the resilience to counter the effects of poverty (Hooper *et al.*, 2007). This is related to social capital which, broadly, refers to the social networks and relationships people have in their communities and 'the levels of trust and reciprocity that exist between people' (Gill and Jack, 2007: 26). High levels of social capital are thought to bring positive social outcomes: reduced crime rates, better health and higher educational attainment. Gill and Jack (2007) note however that social capital tends to reflect the socio-economic characteristics of neighbourhoods: more deprived areas tend to have lower social capital. However, the relationship is not straightforward. For instance, parents who are poor but live in relatively affluent areas can feel more excluded, stigmatized and isolated than their counterparts in deprived areas. And the stigma of poverty can be compounded by the stigma attached to other problems. Hooper *et al.* (2007) found for instance that for BME women, especially Bangladeshis, the stigma of poverty is more intense and is associated with mental health problems and domestic violence. Deprived areas can also be stigmatized, although isolation can be offset by 'the comfort of knowing others in similar situations' (2007: 32).

In Chapter 3 we saw that there can be significant differences between deprived areas with similar socio-economic profiles. Parents' social networks and wider social capital in their communities (that is, the overall levels of trust and reciprocity in a neighbourhood) are important factors in explaining differing levels of known child abuse between areas (Jack, 2004). To illustrate this, Jack cites the example of a deprived part of Bristol, with high levels of child abuse, where parents were 'heavily dependent' on relatives living nearby for social support. Those parents who did not have such support networks 'were more likely to experience higher levels of personal stress, poor health and serious problems in caring for their children' (Jack, 2004: 376). While the specifics of this example are unique to their place and time, it underlines the general importance of informal support networks of family and friends as a protective factor against child maltreatment. It also shows that how such networks function is complex. While most parents in Ghate and Hazel's (2002) study reported generally strong social networks, many had received little help from them. There also seems to be an inverse relationship between need and support: generally parents with emotional health problems, living on the lowest incomes and in the poorest areas, had the least informal support (Ghate and Hazel, 2002).

This inverse relation between need and social support is a form of the social patterning of social capital: that perceived social support tends to increase with socio-economic status. This reinforces the point that if poverty and social exclusion are risk factors for child mal-treatment, then the problem is a societal one rather than one of individual 'problem families' or poor areas. A related issue is how child abuse is defined. A national inquiry into child abuse in the 1990s defined abuse as 'anything which individuals, institutions or processes do or fail to do which directly or indirectly harms children or damages their prospects of safe and healthy development into childhood' (National Commission of Inquiry into the Prevention of Child Abuse, 1996, quoted in Hooper et al., 2007: 98). As was discussed in Chapter 4, poverty disadvantages children in education from an early age and has cumulative negative effects across the life course, up to and including when they die. Seen in the context of the high levels of child poverty that have persisted in the UK since the 1980s child abuse is, at least in part, preventable at a population or societal level: if child poverty was 'eradicated', as the Child Poverty Act 2010 requires, child abuse would be significantly reduced.

As Hooper et al. (2007) note, defining abuse in this way has limitations when applied to practice but locating child maltreatment in its social context is important for at least two reasons:

- First, 'poverty is itself a form of abuse' (Hooper et al., 2007: 98). If, as Spencer and Baldwin (2005: 38) suggest, the 'economic and political factors at country level are likely to be more powerful determinants' of child wellbeing than parents' social capital, then awareness of poverty and social exclusion as what might be called social determinants of child abuse is integral to safeguarding.
- Second, the extent of child maltreatment 'goes far beyond the [number of] families caught up in the child protection system' (Hooper, 2011: 210). If social workers are only dealing with the 'tip of the iceberg' (Parton, 2012), children identified as being at risk of significant harm, measures to reduce child abuse at a societal level are vital.

Prevention, protection and safeguarding

The requirement in Section 17 of the 1989 Children Act for local authorities 'to safeguard and promote the welfare' of 'children in need' marked a widening of child welfare policy and practice, opening out from a focus on child protection, concerned with children at risk of significant harm and abuse, to a more holistic concern with children's general health and development and whether it is 'significantly impaired'. The distinction in the legislation between children in need, an eligibility criterion for preventive family support services, and child protection, is fraught with the general tension between prevention and reactive child protection in practice. Working with limited resources in implementing the Act in the 1990s social workers were found to be '"stretching" the guidance to fit circumstances for which it was not intended' (Sheldon and Macdonald, 2009: 197). In order to be able to provide services to children in need there was a tendency to treat them as child protection cases. The latter would have priority for immediate action but, with resources scarce, other families which required safeguarding were left waiting for services. This is inherent in what Sheldon and Macdonald call the artificial divide between prevention (and family support) and protection.

This tension in policy and practice was linked to social change, particularly the long-term decline of marriage and the 'traditional nuclear family' (Parton, 2011). Historically, the family as a unit had been the focus of child welfare policy and practice but now it became much more child-centred, with a related concern with parenting – regardless of the marital status, or number of parents present. Child welfare, broadly defined, took much greater precedence, with the view that:

> Policy and practice should be driven by an emphasis on partnership, participation, prevention and family support. The priority should be on helping parents and children in the community in a supportive way and should keep notions of policing and coercive intervention to a minimum.
>
> (Parton, 2011: 859)

This new approach informed New Labour policy from 1997, and was tied in with the emphasis it gave to tackling social exclusion and reducing child poverty. The focus on social exclusion, particularly that of children and young people, was based partly on the view that it affects the whole of society, not just the excluded. This led to a more preventive approach where maximizing the educational and employment potential of children benefits society generally because the children are then more likely to grow up to be 'good citizens', contributing to society rather than being 'dependent' on the state. This perspective was exemplified in *Every Child Matters* (Chief Secretary to the Treasury, 2003) and the subsequent Children Act 2004. While *Every Child Matters* was presented as a response to the child protection failings exposed by the Victoria Climbié case, its scope was far more ambitious:

> The priority was to intervene at a much earlier stage in children's lives in order to prevent a range of problems both in childhood and in later life, including educational attainment, unemployment, crime and anti-social behaviour. The ambition was to improve the outcomes for all children and to narrow the gap in outcomes between those who do well and those who do not.
>
> (Parton, 2011: 862).

Strengthening child protection was an aim but 'within a framework of universal services which support every child to develop their full potential and which aim to prevent negative outcomes' (Chief Secretary to the Treasury, 2003: 6). This was a major shift towards prevention as reflected in the *Every Child Matters* five outcomes for children:

- being healthy;
- staying safe;
- enjoying and achieving;
- making a positive contribution;
- achieving economic wellbeing.

These outcomes relate to social exclusion in that they are multi-dimensional, taking a holistic view of children's wellbeing. It thus follows that if children attain all the outcomes they will, by definition, be socially included. The fifth outcome is directly linked to poverty – the *Every Child Matters* 'Outcomes Framework' specifies that children should 'Live in households free from low income' (Department for Education and Skills, 2004: 9).

Every Child Matters built on earlier preventive programmes, particularly Sure Start. When launched in 1999 Sure Start Local Programmes (SSLPs) were a radical embodiment of the progressive elements of Labour's approach to child welfare: a holistic early intervention programme explicitly aimed at disadvantaged children and their parents. The aim of SSLPs was to:

> break the intergenerational transmission of poverty, school failure and social exclusion by enhancing the life chances for children less than four years of age growing up in disadvantaged neighbourhoods. More importantly, they were intended to do so in a manner rather different from almost any other intervention undertaken in the western world.
>
> (Belsky and Melhuish, 2007: 133)

What made SSLPs so innovative was their 'targeted universalism': they were located in the most deprived wards in the country but were universal in that the services provided were aimed at all young children and their parents in those areas. This was intended to avoid the stigma that children's services often have, especially for hard to reach families. Complementary to this the programme was run on community development principles:

> [SSLPs were] 'owned' by local parents, local communities and those who worked in the programme. Because those who benefited would be able to shape it to do what they wanted, rather than it being done to, or for, them, it would not be seen as just another initiative by Whitehall to do something about the feckless proles.
>
> (Glass, 2005)

SSLPs brought together health, education and social care to provide an integrated range of core services:

- outreach services and home visiting;
- family and parenting support;
- good quality play, learning and childcare;
- primary and community healthcare and advice about child health and development;
- support for those with special needs.

Local control allowed communities to complement these with additional services to meet local needs they had identified, 'such as skills training for parents, personal development courses and practical advice and support such as debt counselling, language or literacy training' (Glass, 1999: 258). An inherent problem with area-based initiatives is that they exclude people who do not live in the specific area the initiative is focused on. As an anti-poverty programme one dilemma this posed for SSLPs was that 'by concentrating on poor areas only, we would miss about half of poor children in England who live mainly in very small pockets of poverty in otherwise affluent areas' (Eisenstadt, 2011: 113).

By 2005, a targeted programme was at odds with the universalism of the *Every Child Matters* agenda. Hence Sure Start was 'rolled out' to become a universal service – rather than 550 targeted SSLPs there were to be 3,500 Sure Start children's centres, 'one in every community'. The name changed and, crucially, the centres came under local authority control and parental control was attenuated (Eisenstadt, 2011). This last point is very significant for practice: empowerment, participation and ownership are not optional 'add-ons' but vital if poor and excluded people are to be involved and have a sense of their own agency to change their situation for the better.

The importance of Sure Start, especially in its SSLP incarnation, is twofold:

- first as an effective example of a community-based, preventive anti-poverty programme;
- second as emblematic of the shift under Labour towards safeguarding children, a universal preventive approach to child welfare.

Although evaluation of Sure Start has been beset by methodological problems (see Eisenstadt 2011) evidence that it has alleviated some of the effects poverty and exclusion is growing:

> While the results are modest ... children's centres have been found to be immensely popular with parents and ... they have been successful in reaching the parents who are likely to be the most disadvantaged. The success of SSLPs in engaging and supporting the poorest families without stigma means they provide an infrastructure that is well placed to engage the most vulnerable groups and support them effectively.
>
> (National Evaluation of Sure Start Team, 2012: 7)

What do you think? 5.2: Stigma and self-esteem: accessing services

The quotes below are from two family centre social workers, who work with families with 'high end' needs, multiple, complex and long-standing issues, describing how when families they support are passed on to children's centres, as universal services, stigma deters them from accessing the service.

> Most people we work with, there's an underlying self-esteem issue; regardless of what they've been through, that's a common theme. That in itself is a big obstacle. The thought of going to a children's centre and walking through the front door is just too much. When their self-esteem is very low and they think people are looking at them and judging them, they avoid services, which means their children are missing out on the stimulation and the community activities.
>
> Children's centres provide terrific programmes but they don't really target the families they should. It's supposed to be preventative but a lot of our service users wouldn't dream of going there because they feel that they wouldn't fit in.

Questions for discussion

1 If stigma deters families with acute needs from using children's centres would it have been better, from an anti-poverty perspective, to have stuck with SSLPs which were targeted on deprived people and areas?
2 If you, as a social worker, were working with a family who would not use a children's centre because they felt stigmatized what might you do to overcome that?

Comment

There is no easy way to resolve the tension between universal services, which tend to benefit better-off people most, and targeted services which are often stigmatized because they are used by poor people. SSLPs were exceptional in that they were a high-quality, well-resourced programme specifically intended for stigmatized 'hard to reach' families.

The family centre social workers used two methods to build service users' self-esteem:

- group work as a way of overcoming isolation and building confidence because it brings together people with common problems which they support each other with;
- individual support, including, 'going through the door' of the children's centre with families.

Government guidance on child welfare practice is published in the *Working Together* documents, the latest, streamlined version of which gives a slightly amended definition of safeguarding:

Safeguarding and promoting the welfare of children is defined for the purposes of this guidance as:

- protecting children from maltreatment;
- preventing impairment of children's health or development;
- ensuring that children grow up in circumstances consistent with the provision of safe and effective care; and
- taking action to enable all children to have the best outcomes.

(HM Government, 2013: 7)

The guidance also reiterates that 'safeguarding is everyone's responsibility', so in terms of both what it is and who does it this approach locates child protection within the context of child wellbeing generally. However, while previous safeguarding guidance was explicitly based on the *Every Child Matters* outcomes, in the coalition government's revised version what the 'best outcomes' are is not specified at all. This is indicative of a move away from New Labour's universalism towards a more targeted approach; *Every Child Matters* 'has been quietly but clearly dropped' (Parton, 2012: 157). Moreover, even under Labour's more expansive regime, preventive early intervention was not generally seen as the responsibility of social work which was increasingly focused on protection rather than prevention (Parton, 2011). Following the 2008 revelations of child protection failings in the death of Baby Peter policy was dominated by a 'politics of outrage' (Parton, 2012) with somewhat contradictory consequences for practice:

the final eighteen months of the New Labour government witnessed something of a revaluing of social work and a renewed recognition of the complexities involved, [yet] the actual focus and organisation of the work became even more prescribed and framed by its statutory and procedurally defined roles and responsibilities.

(Parton, 2011: 868)

Shortly after *Every Child Matters* introduced a wide, universal approach to child wellbeing the New Labour government narrowed the focus of its drive against social

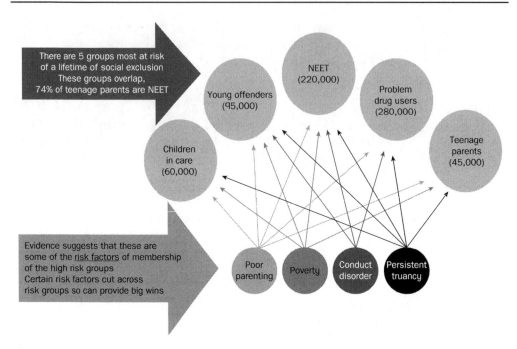

Figure 5.2 'Groups whose problems are multiple and overlapping can lead to social exclusion in later life'
Source: SETF (2007a: 6)

exclusion. After a decade in office, a review of progress on tackling social exclusion came to very upbeat conclusions: that the 'vast majority' were better off and 'poorer groups' in particular had benefited from economic growth and policies which ensured they had a share of the increased prosperity (SETF 2007a). Although these claims were exaggerated (Levitas, 2012b) there was some substance to them: living standards were rising and poverty among children and older people was falling. Consequently, policy became focused on a relatively small '2–3 per cent' of the population in 'deep and persistent exclusion'. This group had not benefited from the general affluence but had 'multiple intractable problems' that could combine and lead to social exclusion in later life. This is illustrated, in relation to young people, in Figure 5.2, which shows groups at most risk and the risk factors which could consign them to a life of exclusion. The argument was that 'cycles of disadvantage' reinforce exclusion, with children in these families likely to grow up to experience similar problems as their parents. This analysis informed Labour's *Reaching Out: Think Family* (SETF, 2007b) programme which aimed to develop integrated working between services to identify families with multiple problems and intervene early to break the cycle of disadvantage. 'Thinking family' required a 'shift in mindset to focus on the strengths and difficulties of the whole family rather than those of the parent or child in isolation' (SETF, 2007b: 4). This was based on the recognition that families were increasingly diverse and the complexity of their problems defied effective intervention by agencies working in isolation: 'tailored, flexible and holistic services' were vital.

What do you think? 5.3: Social exclusion: 2 to 3 per cent?

The Labour government's decision to focus on '2–3 per cent' of people in 'deep and persistent exclusion' is questionable. It was claimed, for instance, that someone living in poverty, with a long-term illness and struggling with basic literacy was not necessarily excluded because if they had protective factors such as supportive parents then outcomes in later life 'are much more positive' (SETF, 2007a: 4). In similar vein, the earlier, vague definition of social exclusion as 'what can happen' when people experience multiple problems (discussed in Chapter 3) was replaced by a narrower definition: 'Social exclusion is about more than poverty. It is about having the personal capacity, self confidence and aspiration to make the most of the opportunities, choices and options in life that the majority of people take for granted' (SETF, 2007a: 4).

Questions for discussion

1 What do these claims suggest to you about whether the main causes of social exclusion are pathological or structural?
2 What do you think might be the implications if this approach was used to inform social work practice?

Comment

There is a strong focus on personal factors and little recognition of structural ones. As was discussed in Chapter 2, definitions and theories about causes of poverty and social exclusion are related to policy and practice to address them. By suggesting that exclusion affects only 2–3 per cent of the population, and linking this to a definition which emphasizes people's personal characteristics, the implication is that the causes are mainly pathological: the fault lies with excluded people. In relation to practice, if someone who is poor, has a long-term illness and struggles with basic literacy is not recognized as being excluded, the implication is that they should not be eligible for services but should rely instead on their own resources such as 'protective parents', which, in turn, implies a restricted role for social work.

Many of the families in 'deep exclusion' are hard to reach, either not known to services or alienated from them. A starting point in trying to reach them is to understand the different ways in which families and services perceive each other (as listed in Table 5.1).

In the practice recommendations about how to close this gap in understanding and so be able to break the cycle of disadvantage, there is a contradiction between the claims of taking a holistic approach and the strong emphasis on parenting, while the wider, social context is given relatively little significance. In this approach – intense early intervention focused on a relatively small number of socially excluded 'problem families' – lies the origins of the coalition government's 'Troubled Families' programme.

Table 5.1 'Challenges of engagement': contrasting perspectives of professionals and hard to reach families

How professionals/service providers can see excluded families	How excluded families can see professionals/service providers
• Reluctant to engage with services • Chaotic lifestyles and unable to keep appointments • Aggressive and difficult behaviours • Lacking in confidence and low motivation • Multiple and entrenched problems mean that they are unlikely to succeed • Easier to refer on to another agency • Poor parenting and life skills • Complex needs or conditions beyond staff capabilities • Need to be challenged more than they need to be supported	• Information on services is difficult to access or understand • Services are not relevant to their specific needs • Staff do not treat them with respect and lack knowledge to deal with problems • Physical environment is intimidating • Respond to single issues without reference to the complexity of problems • Respond to problems when they reach crisis point rather than at an earlier stage • Processes and services are inflexible • Services are fragmented and poorly coordinated • System may focus more on policing than on support – hence a fear of approaching for help

Source: adapted from SETF (2007b: 27)

The research which informed the *Think Family* programme found that in 2005 around 2 per cent, or 140,000 families, had 'multiple and complex problems' as measured by experiencing five or more of the following indicators of social exclusion:

1 No parent in the family is in work;
2 Family lives in poor quality or overcrowded housing;
3 No parent has any qualifications;
4 Mother has mental health problems;
5 At least one parent has a longstanding limiting illness, disability or infirmity;
6 Family has low income (below 60% of the median); or
7 Family cannot afford a number of food and clothing items.

(SETF, 2007b: 9)

'Family type risk factors' were also identified; that is, particular types of family which were more likely to suffer multiple disadvantage. These were families who lived in social housing, where the mother's main language was not English, where there was a single parent and where the mother was young. These factors were called 'parent-based disadvantages' and the argument was that the more of these a family experienced the less likely the children were to achieve the *Every Child Matters* outcomes (SETF, 2007b: 10). As families in these circumstances are very likely to be poor, this is true. However, presenting the issues in these terms (e.g. 'parent-based disadvantage' and 'parents as a source of risk') risks accentuating the pathologizing effect of defining social exclusion in terms of personal characteristics. A related problem is that it tends to take poverty out of the remit of social work intervention – the role of 'frontline' services is seen as addressing family problems, particularly parenting. This does not mean that anti-poverty work is excluded from social work with families but it does narrow the scope for it considerably.

If under Labour 'social work was to operate almost exclusively at this sharp end of child protection' (Parton, 2011: 868) there was in the government's last years the beginnings of a 'rediscovery' of social work. Labour's earlier 'modernization' of the governance of social work, 'with its focus on standardisation, e-technology and performance management' had had the effect of making 'direct contact with families a precarious, time-limited project' (Featherstone *et al.*, 2013: 9). Post Baby Peter, this regime came under sustained criticism which culminated in *The Munro Review of Child Protection*, commissioned by the coalition government in 2010. Munro's final report called for 'a radical reduction in central prescription' with a shift from a compliance culture to a 'system that values professional expertise' (Munro, 2011: 6). Integral to this was an emphasis on 'early help' because, rather than being in tension with child protection, 'Preventative services can do more to reduce abuse and neglect than reactive services' (Munro, 2011: 7). The government's new, much slimmer, *Working Together* (HM Government, 2013) guidance reflects their acceptance of the main thrust of Munro's argument.

While there is movement towards a more child-centred system (Munro, 2012), the general thrust of Munro's analysis has been criticized. Parton (2012) argues that her focus is too narrow, child protection being seen largely as protecting children from 'poor or dangerous parental care' rather than wider social factors. For similar reasons, Featherstone *et al.* (2013: 9) suggest that 'the importance of the family ecology is likely to be marginalised' in implementing the reforms. A theme of such criticisms is that Munro gives little weight to the social context of child protection, a point made strongly by Rajan-Rankin and Beresford (2011) who say Munro mistakes 'child-centredness' for children's engagement with the child protection system, whereas 'Remaining child-centred requires at the very least an acceptance that any examination of the child's needs must involve a deeper examination of the family and community as well'. The Munro Report, they argue, 'is a manager's guide to good practice, rather than a critical reflection on the social basis of child protection, as a concern for everyone living in a "good society"' (Rajan-Rankin and Beresford, 2011).

Anti-poverty practice

Because they are so damaging to children and families, poverty and social exclusion are central to 'the social basis of child protection'. The impact of welfare reform and 'austerity' illustrates this, in two ways:

- first, the number of vulnerable families is forecast to increase from 130,000 in 2008 to 150,000 by 2015, with 54,000 more children affected;
- second, they will be poorer. Vulnerable families are likely to lose on average approximately £3,000 per year by 2015 (Reed, 2012).

These vulnerable families are those that Labour identified as being in 'deep and persistent exclusion' with 'multiple intractable problems', with five or more of the characteristics of exclusion listed above. For these families, escaping from poverty and social exclusion is hard:

> They need a hand to help them take control of their lives and rediscover the hope that gives them the strength to realize that by their own efforts, they can make a difference to their lives. For this group, the specialist skills of social workers and related professions have an important role to play.
>
> (Buchanan, 2007: 203)

The coalition government has targeted these families in its 'Troubled Families' programme. This is a locally tailored family intervention project which has the potential to provide the kinds of support Buchanan alludes to. To do that successfully, however, practitioners should guard against the government's pathologizing discourse (discussed in Chapter 3) which moves from 'families that have troubles, through families that are "troubled", to families that are or cause trouble' (Levitas, 2012b: 5). It is equally important to bear in mind that these are by no means the only families adversely affected by poverty and exclusion. Other families particularly at risk of poverty include:

- ethnic minority families particularly those of Bangladeshi, Pakistani and Black African origin;
- refugees and asylum seekers;
- families with disabled members (adults and children) (Jack and Gill, 2010a).

Depending on which measure is used, there were in 2010–11 between 2.3 and 3.6 million children living in relative poverty (Cribb *et al.*, 2012). It is not then a problem of a small minority and as child poverty grows the need for social work interventions will grow with it. While Parton's (2011) point that the contribution of statutory social work to early intervention and prevention has been marginalized is true, social work is not monolithic but fluid, varied and changing. Opportunities for social workers to engage in preventive work do exist. In part this is a consequence of commissioning and the growth of the mixed economy of care since the 1990s. Social workers are being attracted to the expanding voluntary sector partly because of the perception that there is more opportunity there to do 'real' social work, working more closely with service users and in more preventive ways (Ferguson and Woodward, 2009). The *Every Child Matters* agenda, with the creation of the Children's Trust, bringing together education and social work, and the development of extended schools as community hubs, have also brought opportunities for preventive practice. This, Sanis (2010: 5) argues is 'creating a new breed of social worker, versant in safeguarding children but working on a more preventative level'. Practice of this type has a strong community orientation and is, Sanis argues, 'preventing statutory referrals and broadening social work' (p. 24).

What do you think? 5.4: Domestic violence, family poverty and social exclusion

In this case study of a family consisting of a mother and three children, the mother was now a single parent having fled domestic violence and been rehoused (in social housing) in one of the most deprived areas in the country.

The children were referred to a school-based social worker. They were new to the school, having been forced to leave their home and belongings very suddenly. They were also experiencing difficulties from the trauma of exposure to domestic violence: nightmares, flashbacks, hyper-vigilance and, when at school, separation anxiety from their Mum.

The children are all girls:

- The youngest is 4 years old and will be starting school next September.
- The middle child is aged 8. She is very bright but not fulfilling her academic potential. She has been identified as being underweight by the school nurse.

- The oldest girl is 11 and about to start secondary school. She has no uniform and will have to walk to school as Mum cannot afford the petrol to do two school runs.

The mother is pregnant and has recently broken up with a new partner because of his drug use. She has had several short-term, intense relationships, often with possessive men. There is a financial element to this, as they bring another income to the home.

By an approximate calculation the family's weekly income is £135.30 below the Minimum Income Standard, the amount required for an adequate standard of living (see www.minimumincome.org.uk). The Minimum Income Standard is a measure of relative poverty so the family are very poor.

Their new home is damp. When the family moved in they had no white goods and the house generally is sparsely furnished and 'unkempt': clean but messy because they have no storage. There are no floor coverings and no curtains or blinds. There are few toys and little stimulation for the children in their home.

The two older children often go to school without having had breakfast and never have snack money. The mother cannot afford school uniforms so they have to be provided by the school. She also often does not have petrol money to get the children to school. Nor can she afford the fees for school trips and the children do not have suitable clothing to go away.

Mum has debts of about £9,000. The phone has been disconnected. Gas and electricity are on card meters but the mother often does not have money to top them up. Generally her money-management skills are weak. She says they have always lived 'hand to mouth' so when any money does come in there is a temptation to 'blow it' rather than save or prioritize.

As the family have moved to a new and quite isolated area the mother lacks support networks so the girls are often left unsupervised.

The children had head lice for several months partly because Mum struggles with the demands of treating it – for example, the costs of bathing three children separately and washing bedding without a washing machine. They also have recurring physical illnesses such as chest infections and asthma.

Mum has a heart condition which has complicated her pregnancy. She is panicking about early labour and not having the taxi fare/childcare for the three children. She recently also had a ruptured appendix and was discharged home with no support – the girls were left fending for themselves.

The social work intervention

The social worker works for a voluntary agency and has provided support of various kinds for the family, including:

- Therapeutic work with the girls, helping them to manage the effects of domestic violence by, for example, compartmentalizing/re-telling their story in creative ways to make sense of their feelings and have more control over them.
- Working with Mum around prioritizing the children's needs. She was 'known to social care' when she was a child, is very mistrustful of social workers and is reluctant to ask for help. Because of this she can seem quite avoidant or evasive which, in turn, can lead to crises. This reluctance is because she feels asking for help comes at a price: intrusion into the family's private life.

- The social worker therefore has to be very transparent with her and provide real 'practical' support to balance the care/control models of intervention. She also had to support Mum in contacting the police domestic violence team when the girls' father, perpetrator of the domestic violence, located the family.
- The social worker has twice had to refer the children to statutory children's services for assessment but they have been judged not to meet the (high) thresholds for services.
- Advocacy has been vital, including applying for grants to various charities. An application for a washing machine and beds has been refused because the family had a crisis loan when they were rehoused. The social worker is contesting this decision.
- The social worker has secured other material support including winter clothes, food parcels and toys (Christmas presents, etc.) and Easter eggs for the children. She has also found holidays for the children with charities. Providing this kind of support can open a 'can of worms' in terms of meeting related needs – for example, if she gets places for the children on a summer camp the social worker then has to make sure they have appropriate clothing and other equipment and ensure they can get to and from the venue.
- She has also accessed budgeting and parenting advice for Mum.

Questions for discussion

1 What does this case suggest to you about the relationship between poverty and social exclusion, health and psycho-social wellbeing?
2 What are your thoughts about the capacity of social work (voluntary and statutory) to relieve the family's poverty and social exclusion?

Comment

The family's needs are complex: there is the psychological trauma of domestic violence, the exclusion of having to relocate and the resulting isolation and poverty. All this is clearly damaging the physical and psychological health and wellbeing of both the Mum and her children. Consequently the social work response has to be multi-faceted, providing different forms of support while managing the risks to the children.

Providing material support can have direct and indirect benefits, not least helping to gain the mother's trust. It can also help reduce exclusion and give the children a sense of self-worth, because they see that people are prepared to make an effort to help. Commenting on the presents she had obtained for the girls, the social worker said:

> It was quite telling that at Christmas, both the older girls asked for pyjamas, bedding and a night light – whereas other children have asked for an Xbox 360! They take great pride in playing games and put every piece away neatly in the box. This suggests that they value one-to-one support and also probably don't have many toys and games.

Overall the social worker significantly improved the family's situation both materially and in psycho-social terms. While the family are still very deprived this help will probably have long-term benefits, particularly for the children's wellbeing.

In social work with children, ecological perspectives are widely used because they offer a way of making sense of the many factors which influence children's wellbeing and particularly the interaction between a child and his/her environment. Ecological models are usually seen as having four or five interrelated systems, which Bronfenbrenner (1979 quoted in Barnes 2007: 9) has likened to a 'set of nested structures, each inside the next, like a set of Russian dolls', with a child at the centre. The details of these are beyond the scope of this book but the general importance of an ecological perspective here is that it 'highlights the fundamental role played by poverty in influencing the health and development of children, mainly by its negative impact on family functioning' (Jack, 2000: 713). It also emphasizes that child and family poverty is 'intimately connected' with the social context in which it occurs and so is influenced by factors such as education, (un)employment, housing and access to services, all of which tend to be lacking in deprived areas and which social workers, 'need to actively engage with' (Jack, 2000: 713).

The Common Assessment Framework (CAF) (see Figure 5.3) used in children's services embodies an ecological approach in that assessment of a child's development is related to the environment they live in. Complementary to this, the CAF is intended to facilitate holistic responses to meeting needs by sharing information between all services (via the eCAF database) involved with a family, including adult services. However, Jack and Gill (2003, 2010c) have long argued that the base of the CAF triangle, 'family and environment factors', has in practice tended to be 'the missing side of the triangle' because assessments (whether using the CAF or another tool) tend to focus on factors internal to families, not giving sufficient weight to 'external' socio-economic and community factors. Featherstone *et al.* (2014: 106) explain this failure in terms of the practice context, both political and geographic:

> . . . the Framework ran aground in a landscape of targets, timescales and individualised risk saturated approaches and in a context where child protection social workers were often located in centralised offices miles away from the neighbourhoods they visited ever more briefly clutching forms and protocols.

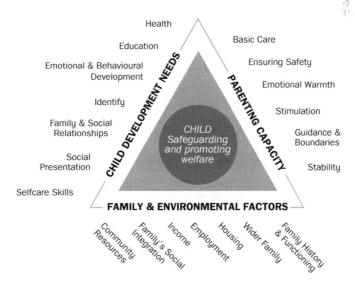

Figure 5.3 The Common Assessment Framework

To overcome this tendency to focus on the 'internal' and the related risk of 'poverty blindness', Gill and Jack (2007: 10) have developed a six-point guide to applying an ecological perspective in practice:

1 Listening carefully to what children and young people, their families and carers say about the balance between the strengths and difficulties in their lives, paying particular attention to what they consider to be the origins of any difficulties and whether they view them as internal or external to the family.
2 Working to make disadvantaged communities more supportive of the needs of all children, young people and families.
3 Working to bring into play the physical and social resources of disadvantaged communities for the benefit of individual children, young people and families.
4 Working with children and young people, their families and carers to enhance their skills in accessing the beneficial aspects of the communities to which they belong.
5 Working to help children, young people and families identify the pressures and dangers of their community settings, developing their sources of support, personal resilience and other coping resources.
6 Acknowledging that children and young people, their families and carers are not the passive victims of the pressures of their situation, and recognising the ways that they actively engage with their environment and play a part in shaping it.

This guide can help practitioners draw out the connections in families and children's lives at different levels or systems. It also emphasizes *empowerment*, helping people gain more control over their lives at all levels: individual, family, group and community. To do this, practitioners need to identify and nurture the strengths which children, families and communities have which can be protective factors for children. In this sense an ecological approach can be a corrective to the negative, risk-averse culture which tends to portray communities as threatening to children because of fears of paedophiles and child abuse networks amid general 'community breakdown' (Jack and Gill, 2010c).

Listening to children: 'empowerment is the thing!'

A social worker describes how she uses a teamwork approach to empower children, using football or whatever sport the children are interested in as an analogy:

> When I go into a family situation I always say, 'We're going to work as a team.' And I include the child in that. I often say to them, 'It's no good if your Drogba's scoring all the goals at one end if the goalie is letting them in at the other end: you're not going to win are you? So we need to work together, we'll do this teamwork thing . . .'
>
> And they just love it, because it makes them feel they've got something to contribute. To say to a child, 'Can you help me with this?' You can almost see them sit up in their chairs and think, 'Wow, I can do this!'

How an ecological approach is applied in practice will of course vary according to the situation. Assessment is, as Rose (2010) says, a relational activity where what the social worker does and how they do it has a great bearing on the outcomes and in which gaining the trust of children and parents is crucial. One of the advantages of an ecological perspective is that it encourages professionals to listen to and take account of people's own understanding of their situation and the roots of the problems that have brought social workers into their lives (Jack and Gill, 2003).

Such an approach is apparent in the domestic violence case study above where the social worker worked hard to win the trust of the mother by understanding her social isolation and material poverty and taking steps to address both. To do this the social worker utilized a range of skills including communication skills, advocacy, partnership working and networking. All of this is informed by poverty awareness, understanding the nature and causes of poverty and how it affects people's lives. In times of austerity, good anti-poverty practice is difficult and it can help to have a vision of how things could be better. As we have seen, ecological perspectives can highlight the corrosive effects of poverty on children's lives at individual, family and community levels. From this it follows that we need, as Jack and Gill (2010b: 93) argue, 'a more comprehensive and integrated approach to the safeguarding of children and young people' than we currently have. Lonne *et al.* (2009: 112) provide an outline of this 'better world' where prevention meets protection:

> Support for children and families who are struggling with systemic disadvantages such as poverty, ill-health, forced migration, and family violence is not achieved by quick fix solutions. There needs to be a longer term focus to assistance . . . [which] needs to come from people being part of the fabric of neighbourhood and community that sustains their children and their families and in so doing builds communities, social capital, and civil societies that in turn grow their own capacity to care for their children.

Summary of main points

- Child poverty, a powerful indicator of wellbeing, is likely to increase in the foreseeable future, creating growing need for preventive social work.
- Child abuse, especially neglect, is linked to child poverty and, in turn, both are related to social inequalities such as class, gender and 'race'.
- The 'social determinants of child abuse' operate at family, community and societal levels. They are not simply a product of the pathology of 'problem families'.
- Safeguarding and especially Labour's *Every Child Matters* agenda sought to resolve the inherent tension between prevention and reactive child protection by taking a universal, early intervention approach to child wellbeing.
- While statutory children's social work has been largely restricted to child protection, the varied and fluid nature of social work generally provides opportunities for preventive, anti-poverty practice.
- Holistic ecological perspectives can counter 'poverty blindness' and help social workers to take a preventive approach informed by a culture of listening to children, parents and communities.

Further reading by topic

Poverty and child abuse

Dyson, C. (2008) *Poverty and Child Maltreatment: child protection research briefing*, London: NSPCC.

Hooper, C. (2011) Child Maltreatment, Ch. 10 in Bradshaw, J. (ed.) *The Well-being of Children in the UK*, Bristol: Policy Press.

Children's and families' experiences of poverty and social exclusion

Ghate, D. and Hazel, N. (2002) *Parenting in Poor Environments: stress, support and coping*, London: Jessica Kingsley.

Hooper, C., Gorin, S., Cabral, C. and Dyson, C. (2007) *Living with Hardship 24/7: the diverse experiences of families in poverty in England*, London: The Frank Buttle Trust.

Social work with poor and excluded children and families

Jack, G. and Gill, O. (2010) The Role of Communities in Safeguarding Children and Young People, *Child Abuse Review*, 19, 82–96.

Parton, N. (2011) Child Protection and Safeguarding in England: changing and competing conceptions of risk and their implications for social work, *British Journal of Social Work*, 41.5, 854–75.

Rogowski, S. (2013) *Critical Social Work with Children and Families: theory, context and practice*, Bristol: Policy Press.

6 Old age: a new social divide?

Key messages

- Ageism is major cause of social exclusion among older people.
- This is compounded by class, ethnic and gender inequalities which consign many older people, mostly women, to severe poverty and isolation.
- Alongside this social divide is the residualization of social care which restricts access to services and puts ability to pay before need.
- Although care management restricts social workers' capacity to support older people, they do nonetheless have a key role to play in combating the social exclusion of poor older people.

> With older people, we find that quite a lot of their social networks have passed away and they're quite often the [only] ones that are left . . . It's a sense of social isolation: I don't think we welcome older people into our lives, I don't think society does – doesn't value them. Even people who do have the means, the money, there's a general feeling that they're not wanted. So the only places they can access are day centres, often with people with the same problems as them and often with dementia and memory problems.

As this quote from a social worker in an older people's team suggests, ageism – discrimination against older people based on their age – is a major cause of their social exclusion. Ageism is, however, bound up with other social divisions. While ageism feeds divisions between older and younger generations; there is also a growing divide among older people themselves. Broadly, this is a fissure between a poor and excluded minority and a majority who have benefited from rising living standards. This polarization is related to other social divisions, discussed in this book, of 'class', ethnicity and especially gender; the feminization of poverty being particularly stark among older people. These inequalities are mirrored in social care, with poor older people having very restricted access to often inferior services. While care management has restricted social workers' capacity to challenge this exclusion, there is growing recognition of a need for a more collective response to older people's poverty and exclusion. Social workers, this chapter argues, have the skills, knowledge and values to play a vital role in this.

It may seem an obvious point to make but poverty and social exclusion among older people is closely related to age. Kneale (2012) argues that social exclusion and ageing are 'intimately twined'; for instance, major life events which are linked to ageing – for example, retirement, widowhood or loss of health – often result in loss of independence and autonomy. From this it follows that 'As people age, their chances of becoming socially excluded are higher than their chances of moving out of exclusion or becoming less excluded' (Kneale, 2012: 102). The same is true of poverty and to a large extent this is because of how older people are thought of and treated: 'Much policy and practice still frames older people in terms of being a burden, a problem to be solved, denied rights to the ordinary things in life because of the processes of ageing' (Joseph Rowntree Foundation, 2004: 5).

This way of seeing older people reflects wider social attitudes and is of course discriminatory. The widespread perception of older people as a burden helps explain the underfunding of services which, with the casualization of the workforce in residential care, is a factor in the increase in reported abuse of older people. Among the practice implications of this, discussed in this chapter, is that:

> social services have become a residual provision for poorer people . . . the process of assessment undertaken by professional social workers is based primarily on means rather than need . . . the costs of care in later life have increasingly been shifted away from the state onto service users themselves. Older people, particularly older women, are being financially penalized for needing care and support in later life.
>
> (Johnson, 2002: 748)

'Processes of ageing' are socially constructed and so unfold in different ways in different cultures. The increased risk of poverty that comes with old age could be avoided. Similarly the notion that as people approach the end of their lifespans they become a burden is largely a western idea. Elsewhere in the world, in Asia and Africa, older people often have status as figures of wisdom and authority in cultures where extended families and reciprocity within families is valued more than in the White, western nuclear family model. While many, usually female, relatives do take on major caring roles there is not the general societal view of respect for and obligation to elders that exists in other parts of the world. As Sheldon and MacDonald (2009: 339) suggest, within the modern nuclear family which 'revolves around one or two adults working relentlessly to pay increasingly high housing, fuel, living and childcare costs' there might not be a lot of space for caring for 'dependent', ageing relatives. The view of older people as a burden is also related to the themes of the 'Broken Britain'/'social evils' debate (discussed in Chapter 4): individualism, consumerism and a decline of community. Being and staying independent is very much part of the zeitgeist as are attacks on 'dependency culture' which carry the implication that dependence is to be avoided at all costs.

There are great variations in how older people experience social exclusion. An SEU (2006) report featured 'pen-pictures' matching different forms of exclusion to characteristics typical of people likely to experience them (see Figure 6.1). These pictures illustrate intersectionality (discussed in Chapter 3): older people's circumstances vary according to a multiplicity of factors, including their previous life history. Awareness of such variations should underpin anti-oppressive practice.

If older people are diverse in their social characteristics, the needs that may bring social workers into their lives are equally varied. As in any age group, older people:

> have a range and variety of physical, sensory, mental health, substance misuse and/or learning difficulties, in different mixes, which interact with each other, and with acute and chronic health conditions, to produce a wide variety of obstacles to ordinary living, social inclusion and the exercise of their human and civil rights.
>
> (Statham, 2005 quoted Kerr et al., 2005: 22)

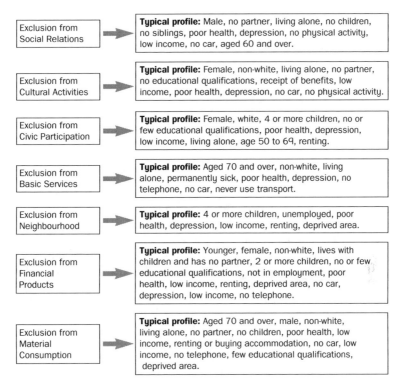

Figure 6.1 Social exclusion of older people: forms and likely characteristics

Source: SEU (2006: 20)

Sensitivity to service users' and carers' individual circumstances should not blind us to the entrenched social inequalities whose impact over the life course can result in social exclusion in old age. Class, ethnicity and especially gender are all significant here, as is neighbourhood: where people live. All of these factors are related to social inequality. Just as the risks of social exclusion and poverty increase with age, there are growing divisions among older people. Most older people are not socially excluded (SEU, 2006) and rates of poverty among pensioners have fallen dramatically (see below). These contradictory trends result in the spectacle of older men (middle class and White) fronting television programmes to complain about having more money than they need (Channel 4, 2013) while simultaneously 1 in 10 older people are malnourished (Smedley, 2013). It is the people who are scraping by on inadequate diets that social workers are more likely to engage with, and their poverty has consequences for practice goals like empowerment and choice:

> For the wealthy, dependency on paid help is a simple fact of life and not associated with any shame or sense of being a burden . . . The choice about whether to go into a care home is genuine for the wealthy – it may even be a prospect to be relished . . . [but for the poor] The abhorrence of dependency, inextricably linked with a fear of loss of autonomy and of being seen as a burden, features strongly in conversations between social workers and older people.
>
> (Lloyd, 2006: 1183)

Ageism and the ageing society

We are all getting older; people are now living nearly twice as long as they did 100 years ago. In 2010 average life expectancy for a newborn baby boy was 79 years and for a baby girl 83 years (ONS, 2012a). While such averages do mask inequalities, generally people are living longer, healthier lives. A corollary of this is that there are relatively more older people in the population than there once were. In 1985, 15 per cent of the UK population was aged 65 and over; by 2035 it is projected that this age group will form nearly a quarter (23 per cent) of the population (ONS, 2012b).

These statistics summarize a major social change which has many dimensions. One immediately apparent shift is that nowadays most people can expect to live for many years beyond what were until recently the retirement ages of 60 (for women) and 65 (for men). However it is, as Ray and Phillips (2012) say, vital that social workers take a critical perspective on such changes. Although alarmist terms like 'demographic time bomb' are often used about the ageing society, the social implications of the statistics do not speak for themselves and are not fixed. A major concern is about the affordability of meeting increasing health and social care needs as more people live to age 85 and beyond. The onset of disability is linked to age and is particularly marked for this age group, the 'oldest old', about 40 per cent of whom are severely disabled (Falkingham et al., 2010). They are the fastest growing group of older people, projected to increase from 1.4 million in 2010 to 3.5 million by 2035, 5 per cent of the UK population (ONS 2012b). The consequent increased need for long-term care is often seen as presenting many problems, about inequalities in access to and the quality of care, both of which are linked to the underlying question of affordability: can society afford to pay for the care that will be needed? By one estimate, the cost of long-term care will quadruple from £12.9 billion in 2000 to £53.9 billion in 2051, a figure which does not take account of any improvements in the quality of care provided (Hirsch, 2006). If meeting this growing need is presented as unaffordable, particularly in times of 'austerity', this can reinforce the idea that older people are a burden on society and so perpetuate social exclusion (Age UK, 2012).

The way the ageing population is discussed and presented in the media reveals much about societal attitudes to older people. Recently, the 'baby boomer' generation, people born in the post-Second World War surge in the birth rate who are now in their sixties and seventies, have been criticized for supposedly taking an unfair share of resources, compared to younger people. For instance, in response to a 2011 report that people who are young now will, when they reach age 65, be 25 per cent worse off than their parents currently are, one BBC journalist described the baby boomers as part of the 'most selfish generation in history' (Paxman, 2011).

What do you think? 6.1: A demographic time bomb?

Put the phrase 'old-age time bomb' into a search engine and briefly scan some of the hits you get. What do the results suggest to you about media presentations of the ageing population? Do you think portraying older people in these ways accurately reflects how most people think about them? How do you think you would feel if you were an older person and were regularly confronted with these sort of messages?

While there is no escaping the fact that the ageing society does have implications for public expenditure, what these will be in the long term is by no means certain. The Wanless Report (2006) on *Securing Good Care for Older People* examined three scenarios for the development of social care. The third was the most expensive but offered a higher level of care with 'improved social inclusion outcomes and a broader sense of well-being' (Wanless, 2006: xxvi). There are options: we can choose whether to continue with inequality and unmet need or to provide better services. What is done about this, what is deemed to be affordable and appropriate, will partly depend on how we think about older people: do we value them or are they a burden society can ill afford?

One cause of growing need is that at present the increase in healthy life expectancy (years free of illness and disability) is not keeping up with the increase in overall life expectancy, so, for many people, living longer also means living longer with a disability. The causes of this are complex but are related to social factors, including inequalities in health (Age UK, 2012). If social circumstances allow some people to enjoy a relatively healthy old age there is no objective reason why all people should not benefit from similar circumstances.

There is no inevitable 'demographic time bomb' or 'grey tsunami'. Population ageing is a global phenomenon, a consequence of the 'demographic transition', a change from a time of high birth rates and high mortality rates, giving a relatively young population, to one of low fertility and death rates, which results in an older population. This is linked to industrialization, rising living standards and improved public health. In affluent western societies it is happening much more gradually than in developing countries and, austerity notwithstanding, in the West generally we have more resources to meet the costs. It is telling in itself that what is a remarkable social advance, that people are living longer, healthier lives, is often presented in such negative terms. The problem here is not the ageing population but ageism, 'a process of systematic stereotyping of, and discrimination against, people because they are old, just as racism and sexism accomplish this for skin colour and gender' (Bytheway, 1987 quoted in Tanner and Harris, 2007: 30).

Ageism is not simply an individual prejudice which some people have and some do not. Rather, it is an ideology which works at a societal level to legitimize the social exclusion, poverty and 'othering' of older people (Tanner and Harris, 2007). A 2008 survey found that in Europe ageism is the most widely experienced form of discrimination, more common than sexism, racism and disablism, for instance. It is also worth noting that young people can also be the victims of age discrimination, and negative attitudes towards young people are particularly high in this country (Age UK, 2011).

Social work, in policy and practice, is not free of ageism. Phillipson (1989 quoted in Kerr *et al.*, 2005: 17) suggested there is a 'tendency for social work with older people to be seen as routine and uninteresting, more suited to unqualified workers and social work assistants than to qualified social workers'. On other hand, social workers have to struggle with the consequences of the ageism of policy-makers who, Sheldon and MacDonald (2009: 340) point out:

> Describe chronically ill older people who need time to convalesce as 'bed blockers' and under the Community Care (Delayed Discharges, etc.) Act 2003 . . . effectively fine Social Services departments if they do not conjure up safe(ish) landings elsewhere at short notice.

Ageism also affects local authority resource allocation, as a social worker in an older people's team described:

> I feel the way older people are discriminated against is unbelievable, even inherent discrimination in the council really: they don't get near enough funding . . . Doing this personal budget review . . . I'm working with some learning disability

and physical impairment cases, not just older people, and the difference in budget and what they're allowed to do is just ridiculous. So some learning disability service users may use all of their personal budgets on social isolation; they might be taken to the pictures twice a week or something like that. But to get that for older people is just really hard.

A common form of ageism is to assume that older people are 'all the same', but class, gender, ethnicity and disability are, for instance, all related to quite different experiences of old age. Bangladeshi and Pakistani pensioners are, for example, nearly three times as likely to be living on low incomes as White pensioners (ONS, 2012c). Equally, what being older entails changes over time; one change is that now, as people live longer, the previously sharp cut off between retirement and paid work is becoming more blurred. Another is that with the rise of the 'grey vote' older people are less likely to be ignored by politicians. This might well be a factor in the sharp fall in poverty rates for older people. At the turn of the century (1999/2000) 28 per cent of UK pensioners were in poverty; by 2010/11 the rate had halved: only 14 per cent of pensioners were poor. Largely because of the introduction of Pension Credits and other reforms, average real incomes for pensioners increased by 44 per cent between 1994/5 and 2008/9 (ONS, 2012c). This is a significant achievement which will have improved the living standards of many older people. Nonetheless there are still 1.8 million pensioners living in poverty in the UK (Age UK, 2012).

Poverty and social exclusion are closely bound up with gender for all age groups – but particularly for older people. Women generally live longer than men, a fact which magnifies the significance of gender inequalities in old age. There are, for instance, three women aged 90 and over for every man of the same age. A related trend is the rise in older people living alone (in private households); and the older people get, the more likely they are to live on their own. Put these two facts together and what you have is two thirds of women aged 85 or more living alone (Falkingham et al., 2010). Another ingredient in the mix is that older women, because of caring responsibilities when they were younger, are likely to have had a broken employment history and so have accumulated less entitlement to contribution based-pensions (than men). Consequently single, older women pensioners, age 75 plus, are often reliant on very low pensions, on average about £50 per week less than men in the same position (ONS, 2012c). This is a consequence of women's life courses: their gendered patterns of paid work interrupted by caring in earlier life, with their greater longevity, resulting in a greater risk of poverty and exclusion in old age. And, as we saw in Chapter 3, old age and poverty are two major risk factors for disability.

Like social exclusion, poverty for older people has particular characteristics. One is that, because their opportunities for paid work are greatly restricted, pensioners tend to remain poor longer. By one estimate, about 20 per cent of pensioners had been in poverty for three of the last four years, twice the rate for the population as a whole (Price, 2006). Another, age-specific aspect is that looking at the range of incomes (high to low), pensioners' incomes tend to cluster around the official (60 percent HBAI) poverty line; with over 1 million people on incomes only slightly above it (Price, 2006). In short, more older people are living on low incomes than the official poverty statistics show and their chances of escaping from that situation are slim. A further implication is that people who are in this situation are likely to have few resources to draw on if they have a crisis. This is compounded by low take-up of means-tested benefits: many (20–30 per cent) pensioners do not claim benefits they are entitled to. The reasons for this are complex but include stigma, the complexity of applying, lack of awareness and access to advice, difficulties with communication technology and language and literacy problems (Price, 2006). Although social workers' direct involvement in income maximization is now usually limited, they should, as a minimum, be able to refer older people to a reliable benefits advice service and, crucially, follow up on the results of those referrals (Foster, 2011).

As women pensioners outnumber men, the particularities of older people's poverty fall most heavily on women, and in older age groups the gender imbalance is greater. Among people aged 75 or older, women outnumber men two to one but, '*poor* women outnumber *poor* men almost four to one' (Price, 2006: 259; emphasis in original). Women's financial dependency on men makes them particularly vulnerable in old age: for divorced older women and those who live alone the risks of poverty are high and, Price (2006: 259) adds, 'many women are catapulted into poverty and much reduced standards of living upon or after the death of their husbands'.

Rapid social change might bring exclusion for older people. The 'digital divide' is particularly sharp in old age: the majority of older people (58 per cent c. 2012) have never used the internet. With services and communications being increasingly online the implications for social isolation are self-evident. In perhaps more direct terms, research into how older people in poverty live shows the nature of social exclusion in terms of being cut off from social norms:

> Inevitably, the pressure to reduce energy costs prompted drastic cutbacks by some participants: one went to bed early to save on power; another reported heating their house for only two hours a day. As for food, participants did not report going hungry, but several said they could not afford healthy, fresh produce. A common practice was not to replace broken furniture or appliances, and a few participants saved money by not having a television . . . some participants had not had a holiday for a decade or more.
>
> (Hill *et al.*, 2011: 6–7)

As the quote suggests, older people are also particularly vulnerable to fuel poverty (defined as spending 10 per cent or more of household income on fuel bills). Some 3.3 million people aged 60 or over are in fuel poverty. This is one cause of social inequalities in health: in the winter of 2011/12 there were 24,430 excess deaths, most of them of older people – equivalent to 200 people dying every day (Age UK, 2012). These deaths are, of course, preventable.

The older ethnic minority population in the UK is growing particularly quickly, predicted to number more than 1.8 million by 2026, a tenfold increase (SEU 2006). Given the high rates of poverty which afflict most ethnic minority groups (see Chapter 3) it is not surprising that they are particularly vulnerable to social exclusion in old age. Nonetheless it can still be misunderstood – Kneale (2012) claims that belonging to an ethnic minority group is not a risk factor for social exclusion for older people, although it is for the general population, because social exclusion of older people in ethnic minority communities 'is largely driven by their increased propensity to live in rented accommodation' (p. 9). This rather misses the long-established point that it is the combined effects of racism and poverty which have marginalized ethnic minorities in the housing market. Living in private rented housing is a risk factor for social exclusion because it is often sub-standard and insecure. Older people and ethnic minorities are both more likely to live in 'non-decent' homes (SEU, 2006). For ethnic minorities, the cumulative impact of inequality which can lead to social exclusion in old age has been summarized thus:

> Black and minority ethnic elders do not enjoy the same quality of life as their peers, continue to have many unmet needs, from care to quality of life issues, which reduce their potential for participation, have witnessed changing family

structures and are growing old in a country that many of them thought they would not remain in after their 'working period'. These experiences are in addition to a lifetime where discrimination and disadvantage have often been an everyday part of their experience.

(Policy Research Institute quoted in SEU, 2006: 102)

For older people from non-White ethnic minority groups the process of ageing is shaped by the patterns of immigration from 'New Commonwealth' countries which occurred between 1948 and the early 1970s. Hence the majority of such older people are first generation immigrants (Nazroo *et al.*, 2004) and their prospects in old age will reflect the inequality and discrimination they faced when racism was more pervasive and acceptable than it is now. This can result in extreme inequalities in, for example, income and health. In one study, while two-thirds of White English people aged 50 to 70 described their health as better than fair, less than one fifth of Bangladeshis and one third of Pakistanis did, a finding which reflects income inequalities. As Nazroo *et al.* (2004: 58) conclude, this matters because older people in all ethnic groups reported 'how their activities and, consequently, quality of life were severely circumscribed by health and financial problems'.

Carers

An integral but often under-appreciated part of social work with older people is unpaid caring. Like older service users, carers are a very diverse group. By one estimate there are some 6 million carers in the UK and:

> There are important variations among this dedicated group of people. 1.5 million are themselves over 60, 60 per cent are women, and there are particularly high instances of caring in some black, minority and ethnic communities (twice as many Pakistani women, for example, are carers compared to the national average).
> (Centre for Social Justice, 2010: 39)

Because much unpaid caring is done by spouses and partners, carers are themselves often older people and thus subject to the similar processes of exclusion and impoverishment as older service users. This is reflected in social security benefits – the Carers Allowance gives the lowest amount of all income replacement benefits and because of the conditions attached to it is paid to only a minority of carers. Not surprisingly, it has been described by Age UK as 'insultingly low' (Centre for Social Justice, 2010: 39). Unpaid caring is also affected by gender inequalities – not only are most carers women but women are also more likely to combine paid work and unpaid caring (ONS, 2013c). As well as the impact this has on their time it will probably restrict their access to benefits.

Carers are also affected by the ageing society; in fact this is an area where the chickens are quickly coming home to roost. The Centre for Social Justice (2010: 195) argues that because of demographic and behaviour change:

> we will reach a 'tipping point' for care when the numbers of older people needing care will outstrip the numbers of working age family members currently available to meet that demand. By 2041 a shortfall of 250,000 intense carers is predicted.

One implication of this is that often unpaid carers will have to do more caring to bridge the gap. This is particularly so given that caring is still undervalued. Thus although carers now have a right to an independent assessment of their needs there is evidence that they are still often overlooked:

> When the social worker comes round he or she generally only asks what needs the person has. Too often, the reply is that their wife or husband does most things and they manage fine by themselves. The social worker then leaves not having asked the carer whether they are able to cope or what the impact on their life is. Of course, the rational thing is to do hide [*sic*] your carer under the bed, meaning that's how you'll receive more support from Social Services.
> (Gordon Conochie quoted in Centre for Social Justice, 2010: 192–5)

That social workers tend to see carers as a resource to draw upon (ONS, 2013c) is partly a consequence of their care management role (see below) in working with older people and the pressures they are under in trying to support people where services provision is underfunded and tightly rationed. But the general over-reliance on carers also reflects their lack of political clout. Carers take on the role for a variety of reasons which include strongly held ideas about family commitment and obligation. And because they are usually the people 'at the coal face' dealing with the most immediate needs of service users they are unlikely to withdraw their labour – despite the psychological and financial stress that caring can involve (ONS 2013c; Lynch 2014).

Neighbourhood

One way in which social exclusion for older people is probably distinct is to do with the significance people attach to neighbourhoods. Older people are likely to spend more time than younger people in the areas where they live and many older people are likely to have a major emotional/psychological investment in their neighbourhoods because they have lived there for a good part of their lives. Thus, perhaps more than for younger people, neighbourhoods can be both an arena for social participation and a source of identity (Scharf *et al.*, 2004). It follows from this that the area effects discussed in Chapter 3 might be greater for older people who live in deprived areas.

Research tends to bear this out, with one study finding that the poverty rates of older people are twice as high in deprived areas as they are for the country as a whole. Scharf *et al.*, (2004: 97) also looked at social isolation, measuring it by three criteria whereby a person:

- has no relatives or children or sees a child or other relatives less than once a week;
- has no friends in the neighbourhood or has a chat or does something with a friend less than once week;
- has a chat or does something with a neighbour less than once a week.

While they concluded that most people were well integrated into their local communities the researchers also found that one fifth of respondents were isolated by two of the three criteria above. It is a sad reflection on the exclusion of older people when engagement with social networks once a week is seen as 'well integrated'.

Loneliness is also linked to area deprivation. In their study Scharf *et al.* (2004) found that 40 per cent of older people were 'moderately lonely' and 16 per cent were 'severely' or 'very severely lonely'. While it is worse in deprived areas, loneliness is high among older people generally, although because it is stigmatized the extent of it might be worse that the figures suggest. Nonetheless the SEU (2006) found 1 in 10 people aged 65 and over feel they are often or always lonely and this increases with age. Loneliness can be extremely damaging to wellbeing; where it results from the death of a spouse, poor social support and physical illness or disability it can lead to self-harm and suicide in old age – particularly for men. 'Social networks suffer as people get older and it becomes harder to make new friends. Social isolation leads to depression, loneliness, anxiety, which in turn stop people from interacting with their local community and accessing services they need' (Anon., quoted in SEU, 2006: 31). In this sense social exclusion resulting from socially constructed processes of ageing can be compounded by area deprivation and decline. Neighbourhoods are not static and unpopular/'non-viable' areas can become scarred by the withdrawal of services and the abandonment of housing which are likely to increase the geographic exclusion of the older people who live in them (Scharf *et al.*, 2004). Post-war immigration concentrated BME groups in deprived urban areas, so older ethnic minority people are likely to be particularly vulnerable to these processes. But it is also the case that older people in rural areas often suffer high rates of loneliness and depression and may be less likely to get social services support to live at home (SEU, 2006).

Forms, causes and patterns of social exclusion among older people are, then, complex and varied. But it can be helpful to think of triggers for social isolation, poor social participation and loneliness as falling into two types, life course events and personal circumstances. These are shown in the Table 6.1. As will be apparent, the two types of factor do overlap and interact.

Some of the factors listed in the table (e.g. decline in mental or physical health) can be triggers for social work involvement but while they might bring major changes to a person's life many of them will not by themselves be sufficient grounds for a social work response. They are however factors for social workers to be aware of and investigate when they work with older service users and carers, because they can exacerbate presenting needs.

Table 6.1 Factors in social isolation and low social participation

Life course events	Personal circumstances
Decline in mental or physical health	Poor transport
Retirement or loss of work	Lack of financial resources
Death of partner, friends and family	Non-English speaking
Experience of crime	Fear of crime
Becoming a carer	Living alone
Relationship breakdown	No local services
Children leaving home	Geographical isolation (e.g. rural, deprived area)
Family moving away	Ongoing poor health
	Gender/marital status – men are more likely to be isolated, but marriage reduces the incidence of isolation among men

Source: adapted from SEU (2006)

What do you think? 6.2: 'Care and control': social inclusion without consent?

In this case study the service user was a 66-year-old Romany Gypsy man, described by his social worker as 'one of the poorest people I ever worked with'. He lived with his wife and carer, aged 64, in a supported housing scheme, after having been made homeless fleeing 'cultural persecution' (or racism) in another borough. The couple were very hostile to social workers so although the social worker did succeed in improving their situation she had to do it against their wishes:

> Him and his family hated social workers and police, anyone in authority. In his property all there was one bed and one chair: him and his wife took turns to sit on it. Any offer of help was resisted greatly.
>
> When I attempted to explain that . . . I could attend a project with them to obtain good quality household items that could/would improve their home circumstances and afford comfort, for example, armchairs to ease with presenting arthritis instead of sitting on the bed or floor whilst the other individual sat in the chair with cold lino-dressed floors – and that further these items could be purchased at good reduced negotiated prices, it was met with hostile verbal aggression and an attempt to physically lash out. My suggestions were perceived as interfering, cheeky even. It was then that I felt that whilst one has to respect their culture that these individuals did not understand how oppressed or poor they were due to their outlook.
>
> He'd had a stroke and had severe cognitive impairment as a result of that – which his wife didn't understand and didn't want to understand. There was a history of domestic violence between them so she had more power now that he was ill. He was also doubly incontinent which his wife didn't understand so each time it happened she would hit him and abuse him.
>
> He wouldn't agree but I improved his life by arranging for him to be admitted to hospital so that his condition could be stabilized so he could go into residential care. He's improved greatly, he's put on weight, his wife visits once a week and they have more quality time together than when they were living together. And he's getting regular food, haircuts, chiropody and things like that. So although he continually says he wants to go home, weighing things up his life's much better than it was. If we'd have left him, the man would have died: he was walking in front of cars . . . His wife didn't want him to go into care because she wanted to keep his benefit money.
>
> Often when they come under the statutory umbrella they are at that last chance saloon really. And although residential care may be something a lot of people dread, for some people it can improve their lives – and it certainly has for him.
>
> There were huge issues of anti-social behaviour in the little complex where they lived. The neighbour next door, who is elderly, she actually had a heart attack [probably] from the threats of violence towards her; the neighbour the other side moved away, I had to work with the housing department, we had to go to court.

> We had to make the changes [without his or his wife's consent]. Its 'care and control': he had lost capacity so we had to act in his best interests because the risks were so high for both of them and for others.

Questions for discussion

1 Referring to the FACS eligibility criteria (see Appendix) would you assess this service user's needs to be critical or substantial and what are the most severe or urgent needs that meet the eligibility criteria?
2 How do you think issues of poverty, oppression and racism contributed to the issues and dilemmas the social worker was dealing with in this case?

Comment

This is a complex case. In material terms the couple were very poor and this was compounded by social exclusion and multiple forms of oppression, not least racism. The service user's needs are equally complex involving an interaction of physical illnesses/disability, cognitive impairment and being a victim of domestic abuse (having previously been a perpetrator). The service user would meet the requirements for critical needs on several counts but the most important is that, in the social workers' view, he would have died if he had not gone into residential care.

This case study is shot through with issues of oppression and power imbalances: the history of abuse between the husband and wife; the cultural/ethnic tensions between the couple, their neighbours and service providers with their related resistance to accepting help. Given the husband's critical needs and loss of cognitive ability the social worker had to act, despite his protests, 'because the risks were so high for both of them and for others'. The case does illustrate the complexity of interrelated factors social workers can encounter in work with older people.

Care management

While social workers should be sensitive to the ways in which poverty and social exclusion blights older people's lives, anti-oppressive practice also requires a commitment to partnership working and empowerment, as this reflection on ageing by Margaret Simey in 2002 shows:

> Peel away the assumptions [of care professionals] and what is left is, in fact, a deep sense of exclusion. I don't belong. I am not one of 'them'. I have no role, no place in our community. 'They' come to do 'good' to me. My relationship with 'them' is all get and no give, a sad and demeaning experience.
>
> (Quoted in Tanner and Harris, 2007: 9)

Older people, she says, 'must be emancipated from their present state of helpless dependency. They must be allowed their fair share of responsibility for their own well-being and that of the community to which they belong'. Simey goes on to explain that the 'clue' to older people's exclusion 'lies in the relationship between those who run the services and those who are supposed to benefit from them' (quoted in Tanner and Harris, 2007: 9).

This raises a critical dilemma in social work with older people: the limited involvement and time spent with service users. This has been greatly restricted by the development of care management since its introduction in the NHS and the Community Care Act 1990. This landmark legislation has had a huge influence on social work with adults, some of it positive but much of it not. A key aim of the Act was to promote prevention by helping people to remain in their own homes and communities rather than receiving institutional or residential care. This was to be achieved by social workers putting in place 'packages of care' to meet identified needs and thereby allowing service users to retain greater independence. The Act also promoted a 'mixed economy of care' by the development of the purchaser–provider split; that is, the role of local authorities was increasingly restricted to being purchasers of care while the delivery of services came from the 'independent' sector, from private and voluntary organizations.

Since the implementation of the Act in 1993 there has been wholesale privatization of services such that, whereas in 1992 only 2 per cent of domiciliary care hours were provided by independent providers, by 2008 this figure was over 80 per cent (Centre for Social Justice, 2010). This promotion of market forces has grave implications for the poverty and exclusion of service users. Although, formally, services are still provided in relation to need, the Act has resulted in the dominance of consumerism in adult social care. Hence, services users are increasingly referred to, and treated as, customers. This is often presented as a way of empowering service users but, as Beresford (2009) argues, policy-makers have promoted a consumerist approach to personalization in which service users are empowered by exercising choice in a social care market-place because they control the budgets which pay for services. This is in contrast to the democratic and collectivist model which originated in the service user movement. One difficulty with this neo-liberal way of meeting needs is that 'customers' are empowered in proportion to their spending power. Lynch (2014: 60) poses the question as to:

> whether a two-tier system will evolve where older people with better resources will effectively have a better range of services and choice, while those with limited resources may have to face the reality of less choice and poorer quality of care.

Unfortunately, this question has already been answered. A 'two tier system' is exactly what one social worker in an older people's team described to me:

> People who haven't got any savings, any income, maybe a very low income, they have to rely on us to support them. And the care we provide, I feel, isn't fantastic. We restrict a lot on what we provide – but if you have money you can have anything you want. That's the difference, there's a lot more flexibility in what you can purchase . . . We only really provide services for critical and substantial needs so if you're not in that banding and you've got no money, you're totally missed out of everything . . . It's real low choice . . . not a lot of choice at all if you come through social services.

Critical and substantial needs are the top two bandings of need in the FACS criteria, the other two being moderate and low, that local authorities currently use to determine eligibility for services. FACS is a rationing device; a way of regulating the amount of need met because funding is limited. Partly in response to increasing need consequent upon the ageing population, local authorities have raised the qualifying threshold for services. In 2006/7 nearly one third (31 per cent) of older people who had been assessed as having moderate needs were receiving support from statutory social care; within three years only 14 per cent were (Centre for Social Justice, 2010). Today very few local authorities will meet needs which are not judged to be either critical or substantial. In a two-tier, market-based system of care delivery a consequence of this is that people who cannot afford to purchase services privately will be excluded; which is what is happening:

> rationing is resulting in rising levels of unmet care needs among the poorest older people in England and Wales . . . there is a growing number of both low income and low asset older people simply falling through the net, people who 10 years ago would have been identified as vulnerable and qualified for care support but now are deemed ineligible for care.
>
> (Centre for Social Justice, 2010: 210)

Rationing and privatization, in the context of austerity and growing need, also affects service users who are deemed *eligible* for services. For example:

- in 2008, only 30 per cent of adults who did meet eligibility criteria reported that they received all the help they needed;
- in 2010 it was found that one third of local authorities had left infirm and disabled people waiting for more than three years for adaptations to their homes (Centre for Social Justice, 2010: 210).

In domiciliary care, the 'quasi-market', or commissioning in-service delivery, has also resulted in the casualization of the home care workforce and for service users the indignities of (what can be) scheduled 15-minute visits with carers who are not paid for travel time between service users homes. As the Centre for Social Justice (2010: 211) reports:

> He [a service user] also states that the rush induced by 'flying visits' inevitably leads to mistakes being made. Sometimes it may just be food left in the fridge; on other occasions the mistakes are more serious. One care worker simply announced, '*I'm finished now. I've got to go*,' and then walked out the door having left the cooker on.

In 2006 the Labour government launched *A Sure Start to Later Life*, a paper and policy intended to apply principles used in children's services to older people because 'Early intervention in later life can prevent inequalities in advanced age and makes economic sense' (SEU, 2006: 25). All too often the services for the poorest fit badly with how we would want older people to be treated: with dignity and respect. But exclusion from services and delayed and inferior services for those who do get them are also self-defeating. One purpose of providing services before needs have become substantial or critical is to prevent or delay them reaching that point. Underfunding and privatization of services thus undermines a key principle of policy and practice with older people: prevention. In doing that, because it most affects people who are poor, what it probably also does is increase inequalities in health. Opportunities to increase the healthy life expectancy of poor older people are being squandered.

These limitations on services for older people are often reflected in the ways social workers engage with them. Care management and tightening eligibility criteria can result in 'formulaic assessments of risk rather than empowerment' (Sheldon and MacDonald, 2009: 346). This can present social workers with serious ethical dilemmas. One social worker described to me the pressure she was put under to do financial assessments (i.e. to assess potential service users' ability to pay for services) following a checklist:

> I feel like I'm being groomed into a way of saying things . . . like 'services are not free . . . all services are chargeable' . . . language is just so important. And people are backed into a corner because we have to say, 'if you don't do a financial assessment we'll assume you have the funds to pay for it'. [Sometimes] people are so anxious that they're going to be expected to pay for it all that they'd rather not have the care.
>
> Plus the caseload is such you've got to get all this information in one visit as well. Now when someone's in a state of panic or stress: you give them all that information, they're not going to remember . . .

In these circumstances social workers are almost bound to be open to criticism:

> Many people's experience of assessments, carried out by social workers . . . on behalf of adult social services or the NHS, is that they are fleeting, bureaucratic and don't get to the heart of people's personal circumstances. They are often used only to decide whether or not people are eligible for professional care, and rarely put people in touch with the local groups that can make a huge difference to the lives of people like Jenny, who as new carers can benefit from the experiences of other local carers and the peer support they can offer in trying circumstances.
>
> (McNeil and Hunter: 2014: 46)

McNeil and Hunter (2014: 3) argue for a new approach to social care with 'a greater value on mutual support and building on existing resources within families, neighbourhoods, community networks' and more emphasis on prevention and wellbeing: 'what it takes to lead a good life'. Unfortunately, they also seem to want to replace social workers (or those in the care management role) with local care coordinators. There is much to commend McNeil and Hunter's argument but this point seems to overlook the complexity of older people's needs and that arguably social workers are the profession of choice for working in situations:

- **'where no one knows what the right answer is** – social workers are [often] better than other professions at handling uncertainty and complexity
- **where relationships are complex** – for example, where there are tensions, disagreements or conflicts of interest within a family
- **where there is a high degree of risk** – social workers' approach to managing risk is at the core of their distinctiveness. Arguably, most other professions primarily focus on removing or minimising risk. Social workers frequently work with situations where there is a degree of risk, but where intervening could actually make situations worse.

(Kerr *et al.*, 2005: 35; emphasis in original)

There is little doubt that social care for older people as it is currently organized and funded often fails older people badly and can perpetuate their social exclusion. There are many reasons for this including structural and cultural ageism and neo-liberal managerialism. Because of this, and however abstract it may be from the immediate demands of social work practice, social work as a profession has an obligation to be more involved. As Lynch (2014: 60) says, 'Practitioners will need to become increasingly more politically aware if they are to fulfil an engaged and empathic as opposed to a controlling role in meeting the needs of older people'.

Manthorpe *et al.* (2008: 1142) show that in practice older people themselves understand the pressures that social workers are under and have clear views about what they would like from them:

> Older people and their carers prized the skills and qualities of social workers whom they considered were knowledgeable about specialist services, persistent, committed, reliable and accessible, supportive, sympathetic and prepared to listen. Thus, a professional and humanitarian approach was a vital element underpinning a social worker's skills and knowledge base.

The Centre for Social Justice (2012: 7) acknowledges 'the unprecedented pressure upon teams of social workers operating in the most deprived areas of the country'. However, it argues that despite the pressure to 'see, solve and shut' cases, liaising with agencies and families to provide care and promote the independence of older people can be both rewarding and worthwhile:

> Many social workers are very aware of how much hinges upon this troubleshooting, preventative role. 'That's the really good part of the job,' one tells us; 'put something small in and it makes a big difference. A 90-year-old can be fiercely independent'.

Social workers' dedication will not by itself overcome the social divisions which often condemn older people, particularly if they are poor, to social isolation. The social exclusion of older people feeds ageism. Conversely, bringing people together builds social capital and encourages acceptance of diversity and difference. In one interview, a social worker engaged in what she thought might be 'wishful thinking':

> I've seen older people cry when they're around children and animals. Why don't we arrange things so that they're not going to sit with people who are experiencing dementia and can't communicate as well as they used to? Why can't we have centres where it's for everybody: all ages, all types, young and old?
>
> (Social worker, older people's team)

This need not be wishful thinking. As McNeil and Hunter (2014: 33–4) show, there are better ways of supporting people who happen to be older, the German example of *Mehrgenerationenhauser* (multi-generational houses) being one:

> The[y] bring together under one roof groups that had previously operated in isolation, such as childcare services, youth groups, support for young mums, day care for the elderly and advice centres . . . These initiatives provide inexpensive ways of joining up various social challenges – social isolation among older

people, time-poor parents and increasingly scattered families – and stimulate the provision of informal care in the community.

Without idealizing such projects it seems clear that they provide a better way of supporting older people than the residualized services many poor people are left with. Having a vision of how things could be tends to make arguments for change more persuasive.

Summary of main points

- Discrimination against older people, ageism, is pervasive in policy and practice and causes or compounds their social exclusion.
- There is a growing divide between older people whose living standards have improved in recent times and those who are often consigned to deep and persistent poverty. This divide is, in part, a product of the effects of social inequalities across the life course which condemn women especially to poverty in old age.
- These social divisions are reflected in the development of two tier, market-dominated, social care services in which choice and quality of care frequently depend on ability to pay. Poor older people who lack those means are thus often excluded from good quality and adequate services.
- These inequalities are exacerbated by the contradictions between growing need and limited resources which result in tighter eligibility criteria for statutory services.
- Although the care management role greatly limits social workers' direct work with older people, social workers' knowledge, skills and values are crucial to challenging the poverty and exclusion experienced by often vulnerable older people.

Further reading by topic

The ageing population

McNeil, C. and Hunter, J. (2014) *The Generation Strain: collective solutions to care in an ageing society*, London: Institute for Public Policy Research.

Older people, poverty and social exclusion

Centre for Social Justice (2010) *The Forgotten Age: understanding poverty and social exclusion later in life*, London: Centre for Social Justice.
Price, D. (2006) The Poverty of Older People in the UK, *Journal of Social Work Practice*, 20.3, 251–66.

Anti-poverty practice with older people

Kerr, B., Gordon, J., MacDonald, C. and Stalker, K. (2005) *Effective Social Work with Older People*, Edinburgh: Scottish Executive.

Manthorpe, J., Moriarty, J., Rapaport, J., Clough, R., Cornes, M., Bright, L., Iliffe, S. and OPRSI (Older People Researching Social Issues) (2008) 'There are Wonderful Social Workers but it's a Lottery': older people's views about social workers, *British Journal of Social Work*, 38, 1132–50.

Useful websites

Age UK: www.ageuk.org.uk
National Pensioners' Convention: http://npcuk.org

7 Mental distress, recovery and mutual aid

Key messages

- Mental distress is, for the most part, socially constructed and so reflects social inequalities. Hence poverty and social exclusion are closely tied to, and major causes of, mental distress.
- Stigma and its corollary, self-stigma, are best understood as exclusionary processes which compound and perpetuate mental distress.
- Social inequalities in mental health are particularly acute for some BME communities, among whom mental distress reflects wider social disadvantage and whose exclusion from, and in, mental health services is sharp and sometimes brutal.
- Service users have played a vital role in the struggle for mental health in, for example, developing recovery as a collective and empowering philosophy which challenges unequal power relations.
- Group work is a key intervention by which social workers can promote mutual aid, supporting service users and carers by working collectively to overcome mental distress.

> Like a dying star eventually collapses under its own weight and becomes a void, my personality collapsed and I became . . . nothing. A walking bag of bones and fat and sinew, moving automatically through the world while the real Tania disappeared somewhere, shrunken and defeated. The simplest of tasks . . . became huge, seemingly insurmountable hurdles . . . I spent my days watching black and white movies and knitting mindlessly. I lost 40lbs because I forgot to eat.
>
> (Brown, 2014).

This chapter explores how poverty, social exclusion and mental distress interact in toxic combinations with often devastating effects on people's lives. In trying to understand the nature of mental distress a useful starting point is causation: does poverty and/or exclusion cause mental distress or vice versa? The argument here is that the causes of mental distress are mainly social and thus that a social realist perspective, which accepts that some distress has bio-medical roots, is useful in helping social workers make sense of its complexities. From this, it is argued that rather than being seen as discriminatory incidents in service users' lives, stigma and self-stigma are processes of social exclusion which are socially constructed and therefore reflect and reinforce unequal power relations in society. The interaction of poverty, social exclusion and discrimination is then explored in analysing the inequalities in mental health experienced by most BME communities. Looking particularly at the experience of young Black men, the argument is that the main causes of persistent and stark inequalities are a combination of social deprivation and institutionalized racism in mental health services. The last but, perhaps, most important part of the chapter considers two ways service users exercise agency in combating social exclusion in mental health. First, it is argued that *recovery* as an empowering approach to mental distress, developed by the service user movement, is complementary to and should inform practice in mental health social work. Second, mutual aid is discussed as a way of realizing the aims of the recovery approach and which thereby provides opportunities for social workers to work collaboratively with service users in, especially, group work. The approach taken throughout this chapter is, following Karban (2011), not to focus on *mental health* as a discrete social work specialism but, rather, to see *mental distress* as a critical issue which occurs in all areas of practice.

Poverty, social exclusion and mental distress

Self-harm among adolescents is reported to have tripled in the decade since 2002: one in five young people (aged 11, 13 and 15) in England say they self-harm. Similarly, the number of children counselled for loneliness by ChildLine tripled in the five years to 2008/9 (Hutchinson and Woods, 2010). The underlying causes of these trends are not fully understood. However, in a view that accords with the 'social evils' discussed in Chapter 4, Professor Fiona Brooks suggests 'modern life' is an underlying factor in the 'ticking timebomb' of worsening adolescent mental health:

> We don't yet know enough about why this is but parents are busy and stressed, and children's lives are becoming more pressurised. They know they need better grades to get to university, but there's no guarantee of a job at the end of it all.
> (Quoted in Bacino, 2014)

It seems likely that poverty and social exclusion are also factors in this. In the early years of the recession (2008–10) there were 1,001 more suicides than historical trends would have indicated, with a large part of the increase put down to rising unemployment (Barr *et al.*, 2012). Poverty and exclusion affect mental health in different ways for different groups in society. A report on the impact of the recession in London argues, for instance, that women's mental health is particularly at risk because 'they are more likely than men to handle family budgets, have caring responsibilities and are often the "shock absorbers" of reduced family incomes' (UCL Institute of Health Equity, 2012: 27).

Mental distress is linked to poverty and inequality in two ways:

1 The greater income inequality there is in society, the greater the prevalence of mental distress is likely to be (Wilkinson and Pickett, 2009).
2 And, as might be expected, it is people who are at the wrong end of social inequalities who are more likely to suffer mental health problems: there is a social gradient in mental distress (Marmot Review Team, 2010).

There is no doubt that poverty and mental distress are related, the question is whether the relationship is causal and, if so, in what direction causality runs. There are two perspectives on this: social causation and social selection. In summary, the social causation argument is that disadvantage (bad housing, unsafe environments, low income and debt, poorly paid and insecure work and the stress associated with these things) jeopardizes people's mental health. By contrast, the social selection perspective (sometimes called 'social drift') is that the impact that mental distress has on people's lives (e.g. in adversely affecting their education or employment) is likely to result in them drifting down the social scale (Murali and Oyebode, 2004).

Social workers do need to understand *why* poor people are more likely to suffer mental distress (and vice versa) but to some extent trying to decide whether social causation or selection is the better theory is beside the point. As the research suggests, the likelihood is that both theories are valid. This is the view taken by the Royal College of Psychiatrists (2009: 8): 'Mental ill health', it states, 'is both a *cause* and *consequence* of exclusion and there are complex and multidimensional relationships between disadvantage and mental illness' (emphasis in original). The blurring of cause and consequence is a reality that social workers have to deal with; for people with mental health problems it can lock them into a vicious cycle of deepening social exclusion as poverty erodes mental health and mental distress increases poverty (WHO, 2007).

The complexities of cause and effect notwithstanding, at a fundamental level the relationship between poverty and mental distress is clear: 'Basically the poorer a person is the more likely they are to have a mental health problem. A class gradient is evident in mental health status across the bulk of the diagnostic groups . . .' (Rogers and Pilgrim, 2010: 51). This close link between mental distress and social exclusion is evident in two frequently cited statistics:

- in 2007 nearly a quarter (23 per cent) of the population in England were found to have some form of mental health problem (McManus *et al.*, 2009);
- only 24 per cent of people with a long-term mental health problem are in work; the lowest proportion of any of the main groups of disabled people (Gould, 2010).

What do you think? 7.1: Mental distress and social exclusion

A survey of adult mental health in 2000 found that:

- adults with a mental health problem were more likely (than those without) to be single, divorced or separated and less likely to be married. They were also more likely to be living on their own;
- people with mental health problems were, broadly, twice as likely to have experienced three adverse life events: separation or divorce; serious injury, illness or assault; and having had a 'serious problem' with a close friend or relative;
- they were also more likely to have had a major financial crisis and to have been in trouble with the police and made a court appearance because of it;
- people with a psychotic disorder (or severe mental distress) were more likely to have left school before age 16 and not have any qualifications;
- a sadly unsurprising inequality is that people with psychosis were more than 10 times more likely to have run away from home (34 per cent compared to 3 per cent for people with no mental health problems) (Meltzer *et al.*, 2002).

Questions for discussion

1 What do these findings suggest to you about the experience of mental distress and the impact that it can have on people's lives?
2 What might they also suggest about the significance of mental health to social work practice?

Comment

The survey results are indicative of the instability and disadvantage that often accompanies mental distress: people with mental health problems are more likely to have suffered crises in their lives, whether they be financial, personal or social. One implication of this is that the impact of such crises can be cumulative: deepening and prolonging mental distress and social exclusion. The case for early intervention, for a preventive approach, follows from this.

A second point is that much of social work practice is concerned with supporting people who have suffered crisis, instability and disadvantage – which can often damage their mental wellbeing. This is the basis of Karban's (2011: 3) argument that mental health is 'at the heart of social work'. Mental distress occurs in all service user groups and so is a practice issue for social workers generally, not only those who specialize in mental health.

The social construction of mental distress

One reason why the relationship between mental distress and poverty is not straightforward is that the nature of mental ill health is itself complex. There is a broad distinction between organic and functional disorders, where organic disorders have some physical pathology (e.g. some forms of dementia and brain damage) and functional disorders are where diagnoses are based on behavioural symptoms. The two can co-exist: stereotypically dementia is portrayed as characteristic of older people but many more older people have depression and, while most older people have neither condition, some have both (Karban 2011).

Functional disorders are generally seen as being of two types:

1 Psychoses, defined as 'severe and enduring mental health problems including psychotic disorders (schizophrenia and bipolar affective disorder, also known as manic depression)' (SEU, 2004: 11). Psychoses are usually thought to be caused by biological disturbances and give rise to 'disturbances in thinking and perception that are severe enough to distort the person's perception of the world' (Meltzer et al., 2002: 86).
2 More common mental health problems such as anxiety, depression, phobias, obsessive compulsive and panic disorders. While these conditions cause great distress they do not normally bring the 'disturbances to thinking and perception' associated with psychotic disorders.

This division is problematic, partly because diagnoses of specific mental illnesses 'do not stand up well as scientifically reliable constructs' (Tew, 2011: 24). And if the main concern is with how mental distress affects people's lives then, as Tew points out, people can be 'completely incapacitated' by 'less serious' conditions such as depression while others, with severe conditions like schizophrenia or bipolar disorder, may have a relatively good quality of life, holding down a job and having a secure family life.

What mental distress is, then, is problematic and contested. This has consequences for the social exclusion, and inclusion, of people who experience mental distress. Like poverty, what we think the problem is (definition) and what its causes are will shape how we respond to it in policy and practice. As a starting point, one definition of mental illness is 'Clinically recognisable patterns of psychological symptoms or behaviour causing acute or chronic ill-health, personal distress or distress to others' (WHO, 1992 quoted in Karban 2011: 31). This definition fits within the psychiatric discourse dominant in mental health services. As Rogers and Pilgrim (2010: 2) point out, psychiatrists '. . . see their role as identifying sick individuals (diagnosis), predicting the future course of their illness (prognosis), speculating about its cause (aetiology) and prescribing a response to the condition, to cure it or ameliorate its symptoms (treatment)'. This is the essence of the 'medical model of mental health' which, as Gould (2010) says can be something of a caricature, a 'straw man' set up as an easy target for criticizing medical-ized responses to problems which have their roots in social conditions. While a medical perspective probably would see the main causes of mental distress as emanating from biology and genetics, social causation is now widely recognized as a contributory factor:

> For instance, a psychiatrist treating a patient with anti-depressant drugs may recognize fully that living in a high-rise flat and being unemployed have been the main causes of the depressive illness, and may assume that the stress this causes has triggered biochemical changes in the brain, which can be corrected by using medication.
>
> (Rogers and Pilgrim, 2010: 2)

Nonetheless, responses to mental distress remain predominantly medicalized and within that there are, as Karban (2011) says, identifiable features of a medical model:

- mental distress is seen as having an objective disease process;
- primacy is given to the influence of genetic, biological and/or chemical factors;
- responses to distress are based on diagnosis and treatment by professionals.

However, the medical model is, in one sense, 'past its sell-by date': most mental health professionals probably now subscribe to some variant of the bio-psycho-social model (BPS model) (Campbell and Davidson, 2012). This is based on systems theory in which people are seen as being located within whole systems comprising both the sub-personal (the nervous system, etc.) and the supra-personal: the wider psycho-social context which can be seen as emanating out from the individual in layers of increasing complexity (Gould, 2010). The key point of the BPS model is that mental illness can only be fully understood by taking account of the whole system. In taking this holistic approach the model should facilitate multi-disciplinary working. But how the BPS model is understood and applied varies. In the example above of the (notional) psychi-atrist who recognizes the social roots of a person's depression but prescribes anti-depressants, she or he may well subscribe to a BPS model but is likely to have a different understanding of it than a social worker (whose priorities might be to improve the person's living conditions and help them overcome their social isolation). Such different conceptions of the BPS model and thus of practice priorities are bound up with issues of power.

Debates about models can be abstract, conducted largely among professionals and academics and distant from service users' lives. Yet in one very powerful sense the medical model remains potent: it still holds sway in public opinion and thereby generates stigma and self-stigma – both of which cause social exclusion: 'The medical model is such a dominant way of viewing our lives that it does not allow for other discussion, and therefore consigns the "ill" person to a negative outlook on life, which is mirrored by society's reaction to us' (Coldham, 2010: 4). The emergence of the BPS model is clearly an improvement on the limitations of the medical model. Yet the continued dominance of psychiatry points to the value of a social constructivist (or constructionist) perspective in which 'fixed and dominant notions of power and oppression are examined for their role in reinscribing systems of power and oppression' (Karban, 2011: 43). Social constructivism questions whether there is an objective reality of mental illness. Rather, the argument is that perceived mental disorders are products of their particular social context and the power relationships therein. The problematic nature of medical diagnoses of mental disorders can be seen as evidence of this. Historically, such diagnoses can be seen as ways of controlling behaviours which present 'a challenge to the status quo, or represent attempts to survive or escape oppression' (Karban, 2011: 43). One historical example of this is drapetomania, a supposed illness which in the USA during the nineteenth century was thought to cause slaves to run away. Similarly, for much of the twentieth century, homosexuality was classified as a mental disorder with the consequence that gay people were subjected to damaging attempts to 'cure' them (Coppock and Dunn, 2010). Both forms of oppression have contemporary relevance. Drapetomania has echoes today in the institutional racism of the mental health system (Fernando, 2010), while Carr (2003: 34) claims that 'many mental health practitioners still operate using the disease model of homosexuality because it is integral to their inherited clinical thought and practice'. Racism is discussed more later; here the point is that a social constructivist perspective can highlight the social control aspects of practice which are often most pronounced in work with poor and excluded groups.

Useful as they are, to some extent, social causation and social constructivism are at odds in that the former accepts the reality of mental illness whereas the latter, implicitly at least, denies its existence as anything more than a social construct. Social realism provides a way of reconciling this contradiction because as Karban (2011: 44) says:

> social realism enables the acknowledgement of the reality of mental health and the social factors which may contribute to mental ill health, whilst at the same time maintaining a critical perspective on the ways in which the meaning of mental health is produced.

A social realist perspective can bridge the gap between some of the more abstract theoretical criticisms of the medical model and the 'real world' of service users' struggles with the psycho-social 'insults to health' inflicted by poverty and exclusion. To use Rogers and Pilgrim's (2010) term, it can help social workers 'do business' with psychiatry while maintaining a critical perspective on the medicalization of what are primarily social problems.

What do you think? 7.2: Conduct disorders

In 2004 a survey of the mental health of children and young people (aged 5–16, in Great Britain) found that 10 per cent had a 'clinically diagnosed mental disorder' and 6 per cent had a conduct disorder (Green et al., 2005). According to NICE (2013: 4), 'Conduct disorders are characterised by repetitive and persistent patterns of antisocial, aggressive or defiant behaviour that amounts to significant and persistent violations of age appropriate social expectations'. The 2004 survey found that social exclusion and poverty ran high in these children's families. Children with conduct disorders, the most prevalent psychiatric disorder among children and adolescents, are more likely to be boys and tend to be older (aged 11–16); they are also more likely than other children to:

1 Be living with cohabiting, single or previously married lone parents and more likely to be in large families (four or more children).
2 Have parents with no educational qualifications and live in low-income families.
3 Be behind with their schooling, have more absence from school, play truant and be excluded from school.
4 Be living with a parent with an emotional disorder (e.g. depression) and to have experienced their parents' separation.
5 Find it harder to make and keep friends.
6 Smoke, take drugs and drink.

Questions for discussion

1 What do the characteristics of these children suggest to you about:
The diagnosis of conduct disorders?
Their causes?

Comment

Gould (2010) warns against a tendency among critics of psychiatric diagnoses to treat conduct disorders as 'dustbin' categories for anti-social behaviour. Yet, NICE (2013: 4) reports that there is 'a steep social class gradient, with a three- to four-fold increase in prevalence in social classes D and E compared with social class A'. As might be expected, children with conduct disorders are massively over-represented among looked-after children, those who have been abused and those on child protection registers.

Thus, from a social realist perspective, conduct disorders would seem to fit with Tew's (2011: 20, emphasis in original) argument that mental distress can be seen as both:

- a way of coping with (or containing) our underlying unease; and
- a 'cry for help' that may also express (often indirectly) what the unease may be about.

Green et al.'s finding that 21 per cent of children with conduct disorders had tried to harm or kill themselves is indicative, perhaps, of the scale of their distress.

A social model of madness?

Social realism can inform a social model of mental health and there are parallels here between physical disability and mental distress in that for both the impact of the social environment can be more 'disabling' than the condition (or impairment) itself. However, applying the social model of disability to mental health is problematic partly because, as Tew (2011: 104) points out, the experiences are different:

> Instead of facing just the 'double whammy' of impairment and socially imposed disability, people with mental health difficulties tend to face a 'triple whammy' in which they have to contend with not just their original distress experiences, but also potentially extreme responses of stigmatisation that may then, in turn, exacerbate their level of mental distress.

The social model of disability was developed by the Disabled People's Movement as part of their struggle for equality (see Chapter 3). Research has shown that while many service users and survivors identified with the Disabled People's Movement and the social model of disability, they also had doubts about the relevance of impairment (Beresford *et al.*, 2010). From this some service users saw a need to develop a distinct 'social model of madness and distress' (albeit with some reservations about the term 'madness') that:

> would help create solidarity and shared understandings between different user groups and improve the chances for joint campaigning. If more service user groups drew on such a social model, then it would be likely to be stronger and opportunities for collaboration would be increased. It could also help highlight the links between different people's distress and make clearer how individual distress might be associated with broader oppression and discrimination.
>
> (Beresford *et al.*, 2010: 24)

A social model of madness could then assist service users and survivors to exercise agency collectively to tackle entrenched social exclusion.

Social causation of mental distress is akin to the social determinants of health: the socio-economic conditions which give rise to general inequalities in health. As discussed in Chapter 4, the psycho-social stress generated by deprivation and inequality is a cause of the higher rates of physical illness and shorter lives of poor people. As this suggests, physical and mental health are inter-related: people with physical ailments are more likely to experience mental distress and vice versa. In an unequal society, socio-economic status shapes inequalities in both physical and mental health. In Friedli's words (2009: 9), social inequality 'structures individual and collective experiences of dominance, hierarchy, isolation, support and inclusion'. This is not only because 'insults to health' are socially determined but also because individual resources which protect mental health, 'confidence, self efficacy, optimism and connectedness are embedded within social structures' (Friedli, 2009: 9).

Life course perspectives can help to explain the socially structured distribution of risks and protective factors in mental health and help social workers understand the varied ways they impact on the lives of individual service users. This is explained more in Chapter 4 but, in summary, a life course perspective allows the mapping of links between children's early life situation and their likely outcomes in adulthood. A life course approach is particularly useful in showing how the damaging effects of social inequality can be carried through a person's life. This can occur cumulatively as, for example, in a child growing up in poverty, underachieving at school and then struggling to find decent work as an adult. There are also 'critical periods' when outcomes can be skewed by inequality to perpetuate or compound it; these include episodes like starting or changing school and leaving the parental home. Either way, for people who are poor and excluded these experiences are more likely to be stressful and may well be detrimental to mental health. Friedli (2009) makes three key points about the relevance of the life course to mental distress:

1 That, because the life course focuses on the psycho-social impact of poverty and exclusion, it highlights the central importance of mental health to children's life chances.
2 That mental health is probably 'a key factor in explaining the power of the life course model in predicting outcomes' (p. 32).
3 That in terms of mental health across the lifespan, the rich get richer and the poor get poorer.

Mental distress in childhood is a strong predictor of disadvantage in adulthood. For example, Friedli (2009: 33) shows powerfully the extent to which conduct disorders among children and young people are associated with social exclusion and poverty later in life:

> It is found, for example, that those in the bottom 5% in terms of disturbed childhood behaviour are four times as likely as those in the top 50% to have committed a violent offence by age 25, three times as likely to have attempted suicide and nearly three times as likely to have become a teenage parent . . . and nearly one and a half times more likely to have no qualifications.

Parsonage, *et al.* (2014) emphasize inter-generational effects, arguing that there is plenty of evidence that children with conduct disorders may later become parents of children with the same diagnosis. There are several factors which might cause this; Parsonage *et al.* (p. 19) argue that as well as a 'genetic component' in the early onset of conduct disorder:

> . . . there is evidence of assortative mating between people with behavioural problems, which compounds the genetic risk and also exposes children to adverse influences in the home environment such as relationship violence . . . [and] that parents with a history of behavioural problems are more hostile and harsh in their parenting styles than other parents.

This appears to lean towards pathological explanations of poverty (discussed in Chapter 2). The emphasis on genetics perhaps reflects contemporary discourses which give genes primacy as 'unit characters': single elements which cause physiological and behavioural traits. This, as Leader (2011) says, echoes early twentieth-century eugenics and 'was disproven about a century ago'; yet still, 'genes are seen as isolated causal agents rather than as parts of complex networks of biological interactions that usually depended to a large extent on what was going on in the surrounding world' (p. 139).

One of the more marked forms of the exclusion of children with conduct disorders is that 41 per cent of them, nearly twice the rate for all children, live in 'hard pressed', deprived areas (Green *et al.*, 2005). As Ghate and Hazel (2002) have shown, parents who live in deprived neighbourhoods are three times more likely (as parents in the general population) to score highly on a mental health 'malaise inventory'. Lone parents are particularly vulnerable; given all the other hardships they face, it may not come as a huge surprise that in poor areas 'raising children alone can be a very lonely and depressing experience' (p. 83). In relation to child abuse, Brandon *et al.*'s (2009: 45) analysis of serious case reviews 'found evidence of many parents and carers struggling with mental ill-health, domestic violence, substance misuse and poverty, often in combination'. This is obviously not good for children's wellbeing; for instance, of children who have witnessed domestic violence, 'over half (52%) had behavioural problems, [and] over a third (39%) had difficulties adjusting at school' (CAADA, 2014: 2).

What do you think? 7.3: The 'toxic trio' and 'storing up' mental distress?

In an analysis of serious cases reviews, Brandon et al. (2010: 53) identified what they call, 'a potentially "toxic trio" of parental substance misuse, violence and mental health problems which often coexist', and which is 'often compounded by poverty'.

In the research for this book this finding was echoed in a focus group discussion with social workers in children's teams, working mainly in deprived urban areas. The exchange below between a group of social workers was prompted by the question, 'Are most of the families you work with in particular deprived areas?'

[SW1] Yes, and they're faced with issues of drugs, mental health, domestic violence and alcohol, they're all entangled together. They feel isolated; they're isolated from their families, from their community . . . [SW2] In quite a lot of the areas we're talking about there's a sub-culture that goes on, and you're not only working with the families, you're trying to counter-act the draw of the sub-culture . . . because the sub-culture is drugs, alcohol, domestic violence . . . [SW3] which is widely accepted . . . because it's the way of life . . .

[SW2] Even with families who want to change, it's very difficult for them because they're surrounded by families who haven't made that decision . . . [SW3] And how many families have you found who have said, 'Just get me out of this place'? They feel that their problems would all be totally resolved if they were out of the houses they're in . . . [SW2] And we kinda like encounter that on a daily basis, do we not . . . ?

[SW4] It's inter-generational isn't it? And if you're born into this and the opportunities aren't there, so you go to the same school as your Mum did . . . and you may be tarred with the same brush your Mum was . . . If the opportunities don't present themselves you're not going to know they're out there; you're not going to be able to get out even if you've got the wherewithal to do that. [SW3] It's about, in a way, people having low horizons, low expectations, because culturally, or generationally, that becomes the expectation. And there isn't the emphasis on education, there isn't the emphasis on self-improvement . . . [SW5] Because the emphasis is survival really . . . [SW1] Often that is the bottom line: you cannot plan for next year when today is, 'Where's the money to put in the meter?'

Questions for discussion

1 Reflect on the lives of the families described by the social workers; what do you feel about them and the sub-cultures that surround them?
2 From a life course perspective, what do you think growing up in environments like these implies for children's mental health?

Comment

The existence of the 'toxic trio' and the emphasis the social workers give to sub-cultures could be seen as confirming pathological views of poverty and social exclusion (see Chapters 2 and 3). However, two themes of the discussion are the empathy the social workers felt for families trapped in these circumstances and their acknowledgement of the structural factors, including stigma, which blocked people's efforts to 'get out'.

In their study of deprived areas Ghate and Hazel (2002: 62) note that children may be 'storing up' physical and mental health problems for the future:

Many of the children . . . will become the 'parents in poor environments' of the future. Although, as a group, the children . . . may be in reasonably good physical and mental or emotional health, our data suggest that by the time they reach parenthood themselves they can expect to enjoy considerably worse health than parents in the population at large.

The life course is used to examine children's likely future development but, as Friedli's point about the rich in mental health getting richer and the poor getting poorer suggests, it can be applied retrospectively to better understand how adults come to be in their current situations. The roots of the depression of an impoverished and isolated older woman may go back to her family's poverty when she was a child. Tracing that development over time, including the impact of gender inequalities, will give insights into her current situation: how it happened, how she understands it, and so on. However, a life course perspective is not a short cut or a quick fix. The insults to mental health inflicted by a lifetime of inequality are socially structured but they are also diverse and specific to individuals. In these pressured, managerialist times, a life course perspective can enhance relational social work but is not a substitute for it.

Stigma and self-stigma

An influential government report in 2004 identified stigma and discrimination as the 'greatest barriers' causing the social exclusion of people with mental health problems (SEU, 2004). An even earlier report shocked even the mental health charity Mind with its revelations of 'the extent to which stigmas and taboos surrounding mental ill-health affect every area of life including employment, housing, parenting, finances and relationships with family and friends' (Read and Baker, 1996: 4). The report came at a time when, under the banner of 'community care', long-term mental health institutions were closing with patients were being discharged 'to live in the community', often without adequate support. A high profile case was the fatal stabbing of Jonathan Zito by Chris-topher Clunis on a London Underground platform in 1992. Clunis, who had a diagnosis of schizophrenia, had been caught in the 'revolving door' syndrome then associated with community care: of admission, discharge from and readmission to mental health facilities. The sensationalist and stigmatizing reporting of the Clunis case (Campbell and Davidson, 2012) may well help to explain the discrimination disclosed in the Mind report, including:

- almost half (47%) the people had been abused or harassed in public, and 14% had been physically attacked
- a quarter (25%) of people felt at risk of attack inside their own homes [and] 26% of people were forced to move home because of harassment.

Clunis is Black and press coverage of the case also gave rise to the malignant stereotype of young Black men in mental distress being 'big, Black and dangerous', the legacy of which still permeates mental health services (Keating, 2007).

Whether intimidation of service users at this violent level still persists is unclear. In recent times there have been major campaigns to reduce stigma, notably Time to Change (TTC), 'England's biggest programme to challenge mental health stigma and discrimina-tion'. However, evaluation of the first phase (2008–11) showed limited success:

> a small reduction in discrimination reported by service users and improved employer recognition of common mental health problems . . . [but] Disap-pointingly, there was no improvement in knowledge or behaviour among the general public, nor in user reports of discrimination by mental health professionals.
>
> (Smith, 2013: 49)

Although service users reported that overall discrimination had declined, the vast majority (90 per cent) had experienced discrimination and identified four areas in which it had increased, including 'benefits' and 'safety' (Corker *et al.*, 2013). What these terms mean is not explored in the evaluation but they are probably related to the 'demonization of the disabled' in which, in an era of austerity and welfare reform, politicians and the media feed a 'constant drip-drip of stories implying [that] vast numbers of disability claimants are bogus, [and] that benefits are doled out without proper checks' (Birrell, 2011). Citing evidence that disabled people are facing worsening aggression and abuse, Birrell claims that because they may not show obvious physical signs of disability people in mental distress are 'among those feeling the coldest chill of this new mood of intolerance'.

More generally, Sayce (cited in Morris and Gilchrist; 2011: 9) argues that social exclusion occurs because stigma and discrimination create a 'fundamental boundary between people who have a mental health problem and those who do not'. As stigma is socially constructed, based on popular assumptions about, in this case, mental distress, it highlights the importance of a social perspective. Tew's (2011) 'triple whammy', men-tioned earlier, highlights the dual impact of stigma both as a social barrier creating disability and exclusion and as a corrosive agent which can worsen people's mental distress.

In seeing stigma as a process, Link and Phelan (2001) argue that stigmatization involves 'labelling, stereotyping, separation, status loss, and discrimination' occurring together. This happens in different ways according to the context. Fernando (2010: 38) discusses 'psychiatric stigma', stigma attached to a diagnosis of mental illness, usually schizophrenia, 'which carries images of alienness, fear, dangerousness, deceit . . . added to by stereotypes promoted by the media, [and] subconscious fears and prejudices of many people'. This example of stigma emanating from the medical profession underlines Link and Phelan's (2001) insight regarding the importance of power imbalances in stigmatization. They explain this with the example of service users who might label some members of a mental health team as 'pill pushers' and apply to them characteristics which they associate with that label, such as being 'cold, paternalistic and arrogant'. The stigmatizing process occurs but the 'pill pushers' do not become a stigmatized group because 'The patients simply do not possess the social, cultural, economic, and political power to imbue their cognitions about staff with serious discriminatory consequences' (p. 376). On the other hand, one effect of stigma can be to further entrench power imbalances between, for instance, service users and health professionals and, of course, social workers.

Thompson's (2012) personal, cultural and structural (PCS) model of discrimination is useful for analysing the ways stigma is generated and how it affects people. Psychiatric stigma, for instance, can be seen as a byproduct of the culture of that branch of the medical profession. Negative media coverage of mental illness, especially the common misrepresentation of people in mental distress as 'violent, unpredictable and dangerous' (Coppock and Dunn, 2010: 11) has its baleful effect at a structural level. At the personal level is self-stigma; the internalization by people in mental distress of prejudices about their condition. Overton and Medina (2008) describe self-stigma as having three effects:

1 Language shift: both 'clients and practitioners referred to clients as *cases* instead of *persons*' (p. 147, emphasis in original).
2 Lack of love: service users reporting that that they did not feel or experience love in their lives. This is related to loneliness and feeling unaccepted.
3 Lack of a life of their own or control: the feeling that other people were making decisions for them.

The exclusionary effect self-stigma can have is vividly depicted by Kathleen Gallo, whose mental distress led her to believe that she had been consigned to 'the social garbage heap':

> I tortured myself with the persistent and repetitive thought that people I would encounter, even total strangers, did not like me and wished that mentally ill people like me did not exist.
> Thus, I would do things such as standing away from others at bus stops and hiding and cringing in the far corners of subway cars. Thinking of myself as garbage, I would even leave the sidewalk in what I thought of as exhibiting the proper deference to those above me in social class. The latter group, of course, included all other human beings.
>
> (Quoted in Corrigan and Watson, 2002: 35)

For Corrigan and Watson, self-stigma occurs when people with mental distress, 'living in a culture steeped in stigmatizing images' (p. 35) accept that the negative stereotypes portrayed apply to themselves. This results in diminished self-esteem (people's evaluation of their own worth) and self-efficacy (people's beliefs about their ability to perform tasks or behaviours). How people respond to stigmatizing structural and cultural processes is not straightforward. In what Corrigan and Watson (p. 36) call the 'paradox of self-stigma', they differentiate between three possible reactions:

- diminished self-esteem/self-efficacy;
- righteous anger: where people are energized by and react forcefully to stigma;
- seeming indifference: people on whom stigma has no noticeable effect.

Recent evidence of the impact of stigma on young people reveals a similar pattern:

> over a quarter of young people surveyed (27%) said that the stigma and discrimination they faced has made them give up on their ambitions, hopes and dreams for life . . . around the same proportion of people said that they had carried on pursuing their ambitions regardless (27%) . . . and that others' negative reactions had made them work harder to be able to use their skills and talents (26%).
>
> (Time to Change, 2012: 7)

People may react differently to stigmatization at different times in their lives. Corrigan and Watson (2002) relate their paradox of self-stigma to different ends of a continuum of empowerment, where people demoralized by self-stigma are at the 'negative end' and at the positive end are people 'energized to righteous anger': 'I was angry that I'd been crazy, but I was even more angry at the inhumane, hurtful, degrading, and judgmental "treatment" I'd been subjected to' (Unzicker quoted in Corrigan and Watson, 2002: 39). Both these points, that people can move from self-stigma to righteous anger and that righteous anger can be empowering are echoed in Wallcraft, et al.'s (2003) analysis of the mental health service user movement. They make the point that people who become active in the movement are often among those who have experienced the most serious mental distress and had the most invasive treatments. If righteous anger is empowering then social workers should be aware that, in Wallcraft, et al.'s words, 'many of those who are currently unable to speak out may be the spokespeople of the future, given enough resources, encouragement and opportunity' (p. 31).

Ethnicity and inequality

The stigmatization of mental distress is often compounded by stigma and discrimination about other aspects of social life. Carr (2003) discusses how homophobia can make lesbian and gay people vulnerable to mental distress, showing that the stigma attached to both can be internalized. Similarly, racism is both a cause and effect of the inequalities some ethnic minority groups are subjected to in mental health services, creating 'circles of fear': 'Stereotypical views of Black people, racism, cultural ignorance, and the stigma and anxiety associated with mental illness often combine to undermine the way in which mental health services assess and respond to the needs of Black and African Caribbean communities' (Keating et al., 2002: 8). Young Black men are particularly vulnerable to the stereotype of being seen as 'big, black, bad, dangerous and mad', with the result that they receive more punitive and restrictive forms of treatment (Keating, 2007). Most ethnic minority groups suffer sharp and persistent inequalities in mental health services. These vary between ethnic groups; broadly Black people are over-represented in mental health services while Asians are under-represented, but Black people, particularly young men, tend to receive more punitive treatment, for example:

- Black African, Black Caribbean and Black/White mixed groups of adults are three times more likely to be admitted to hospital than the population as a whole.
- They are also up to 44 per cent more likely to be sectioned; that is, detained without their consent . . .
- Black Caribbean, Black African and White/Black Caribbean mixed groups are 40–60 per cent more likely than average to be admitted to hospital from a criminal justice referral . . .
- Black men are also almost twice as likely as White men to be detained in police custody under Section 136 of the Mental Health Act.

(Centre for Social Justice, 2011: 5–6)

These inequalities are related to a 'cycle of oppression' (Trivedi quoted in Keating, 2007: 6) in which Black people, particularly young men, are suspicious of mental health services, and the professionals who provide them fear Black people. This results in a mutual lack of engagement which, in turn, may well cause mental distress to worsen and come to a crisis and this, in turn, is likely to lead to more punitive treatment (Keating, 2007). The human consequences of this spiral are tragic, as this testimony from the mother of a young Black man who was hospitalized shows:

I made one of the biggest mistakes of my life when I rushed my son to the hospital . . . finding that he had been trapped in the wilderness. He went in expecting to come out. When they catch a bird in the wilderness they mend its wing so it can fly. They didn't do that for my son.

(Anon quoted in Centre for Social Justice, 2011: 6)

Arguably the 'care versus control' tension in social work is at its sharpest in mental health. Karban (2011) suggests that mental health services can be seen as a continuum with coercion and control at one end and supporting and enabling approaches at the other. Seen in these terms, Black mental health service users are clearly being subjected to stringent social control. The historical roots of this are, as Fernando (2010) has shown, in the close relationship between the emergence of psychiatry as a medical discipline and western colonialism. But, as was discussed in Chapter 3, BME groups are also over-represented among the poor and excluded. Poverty and racism are closely linked and, in terms of care or control, mental health services can be seen as 'part of the wider state apparatus which controls the social problems associated with poverty' (Rogers and Pilgrim, 2010: 58). This of course does not sit easily with social work's commitments to (for example) empowerment and service user involvement. It does, though, give credence to Tew's (2011: 6) point that 'effective practice depends more than anything on developing an appropriate value base'. Tew suggests a statement of values which should inform a social approach to mental health practice, including (in summary):

1 Working collaboratively – to overturn cultures of professional superiority.
2 Respecting diversity and challenging forms of oppression – making a commitment to ensure diversity is valued and to challenge oppression.
3 Empowerment, inclusion and citizenship – enabling people to reclaim control over their lives.

4   Looking for meaning – respecting expressions of distress as attempts to communicate
    something about (e.g.) injustice or 'problems of living'.
5   Seeing the person in context – seeing a person in relation to the socio-cultural context
    they live in.

What do you think? 7.4: Why do ethnic inequalities in mental health persist?

To tackle the over-representation of ethnic minorities in mental health services, in
2005 the government introduced a five year 'Delivering Race Equality' (DRE) programme. To measure progress, there was also an annual 'Count Me In' census of
in-patient facilities. The final Count Me In survey in 2010 found that despite many
initiatives to address the problem, 'there was little improvement in key measures
of race equality, and that in some cases there was a widening of the variations by
ethnicity' (Sewell and Waterhouse, 2012: 9). Below are extracts from a *Community
Care* article (Dunning, 2010) which gives two contrasting perspectives on the
issue: first from Melba Wilson, who led the DRE programme; then from Patrick
Vernon, chief executive of the Afiya Trust, a charity which works to reduce 'race'
inequalities.

> . . . The Care Quality Commission (CQC) concluded that these ['race' equal-
> ity] targets were not being met, but emphasised that this did not mean
> that services were failing ethnic minority patients. It was a conclusion that
> echoed a review of Delivering Race Equality by its lead, Melba Wilson . . .
> 'It is clear that admission and detention rates are not good indicators of
> quality in mental health services,' said Wilson. This is because the fac-
> tors that cause mental ill-health are present more often in ethnic minority
> groups, leading to the higher rates.
>   Wilson and the CQC said reducing rates of admission and detention
> would only be achieved by tackling causal factors such as poverty and
> deprivation, a job for mental health services working in partnership with
> other agencies . . . Wilson's report emphasised that Delivering Race Equal-
> ity had been successful in helping to make services more responsive to
> people from ethnic minorities and in raising awareness among commis-
> sioners of the need to tackle inequalities . . .
>   [In response Patrick Vernon commented that] 'The 2009 Count Me
> In Survey paints a bleak and depressing picture, and highlights how
> the *Delivering Race Equality* programme has not made a significant
> difference in reducing mental health inequalities . . . Several reasons
> have been posited for these ongoing inequalities, ranging from cul-
> tural behaviours and the impact of migration to social deprivation and
> exclusion.
>   'However, mainstream researchers and policymakers fail to acknowl-
> edge the growing evidence and "real time" experiences showing how
> racism, racist victimisation and discrimination can affect the health and
> well-being of individuals and communities.'
>   Everyday racism, fear of racial discrimination and lack of information
> about services are among the reasons people fail to access services when
> they need them most.

Questions for discussion

1 What do you think Melba Wilson means when she claims 'It is clear that admission and detention rates are not good indicators of quality in mental health services'?
2 What do you make of the differences between Wilson and Vernon about the causes of ethnic inequalities in mental health services? Who do you think is right?

Comment

In abstract Wilson might have a point – if mental distress is shaped by social, biological and psychological factors outside mental health services, it is conceivable that the rates at which different social groups use those services might have little relation to the quality of care they receive from them. But this is implausible: mental health services reflect the society they are located in. It is because they are situated in a racist society that 'for many years the mental health system has been hailed as institutionally racist' (Fernando, 2010: 11).

Wilson's and Vernon's arguments are to some extent compatible. If poverty and social exclusion are causes of mental distress it follows that tackling ethnic minorities' high levels of deprivation would contribute to reducing admissions to mental health services. Equally, the persistence of the cycle of oppression is stark evidence of the need to tackle 'everyday racism' in mental health services.

Mental health and institutional racism

The DRE programme was the Labour government's response to the inquiry into the death of David 'Rocky' Bennett, in 1998, who had been killed while being restrained by five nurses in a mental health clinic. The subsequent inquiry found that mental health services were 'institutionally racist', defined by the Macpherson inquiry (into the racist murder of Stephen Lawrence) as:

> The collective failure of an organisation to provide an appropriate and professional service to people because of their colour, culture, or ethnic origin. It can be seen or detected in processes, attitudes and behaviour which amount to discrimination through unwitting prejudice, ignorance, thoughtlessness and racist stereotyping which disadvantage minority ethnic people.
>
> (Quoted in Fernando, 2010: 11).

A key point about institutional racism is that it helps to explain how organizations can be racist in practice, procedures and outcomes, irrespective of the values of individual practitioners. Fernando draws out the implications of this for psychiatry:

a) Failure by most professionals . . . whatever their ethnicity, to allow for racial bias in practice and institutional racism in the delivery of services
b) Institutional practices, such as mental health assessments and risk assessments that are inherently institutionally racist being put through in a colour blind fashion that does not allow for bias

c) Social pressures that apply differently to people from BME communities not
    being picked up on so that, for example, justified anger arising from racism in
    society is not taken into the equation when mental health assessments are made

d) The sense of alienation felt by many people from BME communities being
    interpreted as a sign of illness – often seen as *their problem*, rather than as a
    problem for society as a whole.

(Fernando 2010: 73, emphasis in original)

Social workers' commitment to anti-oppressive practice does not necessarily insulate
them from the effects of institutional racism. Fernando (2010: 11) cites research showing
that although social workers in mental health teams knew from their training that racist
stereotyping was a major factor in police involvement in admissions of Black people, this
'had no effect on their day-to-day practice'. This, Fernando suggests, was because the
practice culture they worked in was racist. This underlines Tew's (2011) argument about
the centrality of values in mental health social work. Where service users are being
oppressed, social workers have an obligation to challenge this and make explicit their
differences with dominant organizational cultures and working practices. In medically
oriented settings this can be hard and requires skill and judgement (which can be learned).
Arguing for a social perspective and the values it entails should, as Tew (2011: 9) says, 'be
within the spirit of an inclusive dialogue'. The aim is not to disprove medical perspectives
but to improve practice for the benefit of service users.

Values are crucial but social causation takes us back to the socio-economic inequalities that underlie the inequalities in mental health, particularly of Black young men.
African-Caribbean boys are three times more likely to be excluded from school than
White boys (Keating, 2007) and, in 2011/12, nearly half of Black young people were unemployed (47 per cent), more than double the rate for White youth (20 per cent). There is
evidence of a life course effect here too: unemployment among Black males remains at
two to three times the rate for White men, through to retirement age (Hough, 2013). While
the focus here has been on Black people's experiences, it should be borne in mind that for
BME communities generally 'Inequalities are reflected across all indices of economic and
social well-being' (Keating, 2007: 3) and these are reflected, in different ways, in inequalities in mental health.

Recovery: an empowering philosophy

In recent years 'recovery' has become a prominent theme in mental health policy documents and practice guidance. The second of six commitments in the coalition government's mental health strategy *No Health Without Mental Health* (Department of Health,
2011: 6) is that 'More people with mental health problems will recover', meaning that:

> More people who develop mental health problems will have a good quality of
> life – greater ability to manage their own lives, stronger social relationships, a
> greater sense of purpose, the skills they need for living and working, improved
> chances in education, better employment rates and a suitable and stable place
> to live.

(Department of Health, 2011: 2)

In other words, recovery is a way out of social exclusion – albeit that *No Health Without
Mental Health* is another coalition policy document in which the term 'social exclusion' is

conspicuous by its absence. Like much else in mental health, recovery is a contested concept with different meanings which, broadly, correspond to either medical or social perspectives. From a medical perspective, recovery is concerned with treatment and 'often equated with cure, a return to how things were before the illness or injury occurred, a process of getting back to normal' (CSIP *et al.*, 2007: 3). One problem with this is that for many, particularly people who suffer severe mental distress, cure and a return to 'how things were before' may well be unattainable. Consequently, it is more common for recovery to be concerned with how people live with mental distress (rather than cure). For example:

> The recovery model is a framework or guiding principle that focuses on working with the individual service user to identify their strengths and build resilience. It also focuses on working with individuals to regain control, support recovery, and to lead a life meaningful to them after experiencing a serious mental illness. It is not just about treating or managing their symptoms.
> Recovery does not always mean complete recovery from a mental health problem. For many people, it is about staying in control of their life despite their mental health problem.
>
> (SCIE, 2012: 3)

The definition used in *No Health Without Mental Health* describes recovery as 'A deeply personal, unique process of changing one's attitudes, values, feelings, goals skills and/or roles' (Anthony, 1993, quoted in Department of Health, 2011: 90). There is an implicit contradiction here in that if mental distress and the social exclusion which accompanies it are socially caused, can they be addressed by models of recovery which are couched in such individualistic terms?

Recovery was pioneered by the international service user movement from the 1970s, beginning in the USA. It 'represents a significant challenge to the status quo and the power imbalance between service users and mental health professionals' (McDermott, 2014: 68). O'Hagan describes how the service user movement in New Zealand 'redefined' recovery, moving away from individualistic American interpretations:

> New Zealand is one of the few western countries that has seriously attempted to right the wrongs of white colonialism . . . and we needed to acknowledge cultural diversity and a connection to one's own culture as a key to recovery . . . Again, we wanted to emphasise citizenship and the breaking down of stigma and discrimination as central to recovery. An emphasis on social as well as personal responsibility for recovery . . . fit[s] New Zealand's traditions of egalitarianism and collective responsibility . . . So we put the spotlight on human rights, advocacy and on service user partnerships with professionals at all levels . . .
>
> (O'Hagan, 2002: 2)

O'Hagan sees recovery as a philosophy (rather than a model), meaning 'a set of beliefs that guides the moral value we ascribe to what people do' (2012: 167). This has at least two practical implications for social work. First, as McDermott (2014) points out, politicians have a tendency to adopt progressive language, like recovery, but do so without subscribing to the values behind it. Consequently, advocating recovery does not prevent the government from introducing policies which undermine it, for example:

> Whilst access to decent and affordable housing is also identified by the [*No Health Without Mental Health*] strategy as an important factor in mental health

the latest Department for Work and Pensions' impact assessment on their own benefit changes finds that 310,000 people are at risk of losing their homes. Investment in social housing has halved since 2010 . . .

(NSUN, 2012: 3)

'Austerity' demands that now, more than ever, social workers take a critical view of seemingly progressive policies. The second implication of recovery as a philosophy is for radically different power relations between professionals and service users. This involves professionals making their expertise and resources available to service users while recognizing them as equal partners who are 'experts by experience', people who have gained 'experiential knowledge' from their first-hand experience of mental distress. For this relationship to work it must be 'based on openness, trust and honesty' (Shepherd *et al.*, 2008: 3).

Tew *et al.* (2011: 445) have developed a framework of five interrelated recovery processes:

1 empowerment and reclaiming control over one's life;
2 rebuilding positive personal and social identities (including dealing with the impact of stigma and discrimination);
3 connectedness (including both personal and family relationships, and wider aspects of social inclusion);
4 hope and optimism about the future;
5 finding meaning and purpose in life.

Hence this framework is social in character, giving priority to empowerment, relationships and social inclusion over treatment of symptoms. Tew *et al.* (2011: 445) argue that it 'offers a vision as to the positive role that social work could play within a modern recovery-oriented mental health service'. To realize this vision, they warn that social work must move away from the reactive and individualistic practice which is predominant in, especially, statutory social work and move towards 'a twintrack approach that involves not just direct work with service users, but also developmental work with families, social systems and communities' (p. 456). This should include supporting mutual aid.

Mutual aid and group work

The development of the service user/survivor movement in mental health tends to be seen as mainly concerned with service user participation or involvement in services. In fact, mutual aid is 'the wellspring and backbone of both the carers and service user movements' (Munn-Giddings and McVicar, 2006: 33) Wallcraft *et al.*'s (2003) survey of the service user movement confirms this, showing that the main activity of the movement is self-help and mutual aid. The terms self-help and mutual aid tend to be used interchangeably and self-help is often used in an individualistic sense. Here I follow Steinberg's definition of mutual aid (and collective self-help) as a process through which people:

1 develop collaborative, supportive, and trustworthy relationships;
2 identify and use existing strengths and/or to develop new ones;
3 work together toward individual and/or collective psychosocial goals.

(Steinberg, 2010, quoted in Hyde, 2013: 45)

Mutual aid in mental health is complementary to O'Hagan's (2002) view of recovery as a collective process, as testimony from service user groups shows:

> The self-help is tremendous for people, watching people grow up through it, coming along feeling thoroughly demoralised just out of hospital and thinking that they're good for nothing and feeling dreadful about themselves, doing a bit of voluntary work with us, gradually taking on responsibility, and then ending up going off benefits and working for us.
>
> (Anon. quoted in Wallcraft *et al.*, 2003: 16)

Mutual aid takes different forms. Here the focus is on self-help groups, while the wider use of mutual aid as a response to social exclusion is discussed in Chapter 8. Mutual aid groups are defined as being:

> made [up] of people who have personal experience of the same problem or life situation, either directly or through their family or friends. Sharing experiences enables them to give each other a unique quality of mutual support and to pool practical information and ways of coping. Groups are run by and for their members.
>
> (Self Help Nottingham, 2000 quoted in Munn-Giddings and McVicar, 2006: 27)

The 'unique quality' refers to aspects of mutual aid which are not available from formal, professionally run, services. One such quality is that self-help groups are a way of overcoming isolation and providing safe places where people can talk openly:

> When I came into contact with other survivors, it was the turning point of my life ... I had a chance to talk about the anger, and have those feelings validated. I felt safe to talk about my experiences without being told I was stupid or sick.
>
> (Pembroke, 1996: 171)

Another unique aspect of mutual aid is experiential knowledge, which is different in nature from professional 'expertise' because it is learned from direct experience. Munn-Giddings and McVicar (2006) argue that experiential knowledge in mutual aid is based on collective as opposed to individual narratives and includes both emotional and practical support. Complementary to this is reciprocity: group members gain from the experiential knowledge of others in the group and offer support in return. In their study of carers' self-help groups, Munn-Giddings and McVicar found that this 'feeling of giving something back' was central.

Mutual aid groups tend to be of two types; some focus on the emotional and practical experiences of living with the shared situation (mental distress) which brings the group together, others adopt a more campaigning role, seeking changes in services, or taking on advocacy. These activities are complementary and can overlap. This seems to be the case in relation to ethnic inequalities in mental health, where BME communities face restricted access to services:

> While some community-led groups remain small and informal, others acquire a formal presence by campaigning for better public services or delivering services themselves. They fill the gaps left by public services or operate as complementary to them ... Initiatives run by black groups facing racism and cultural ignorance often address deep distress within their communities.
>
> (Seebohm *et al.*, 2012: 477)

An example of this is Nyabingi, a user-led organization in Luton run by people from African and Caribbean backgrounds with mental health problems. Nyabingi runs a range of activities including a women's support group but, 'The essence of Nyabingi is the way it enables service users, the Black community and wider society to tackle stigma and exclusion' (Nyabingi, 2011: 4). In doing this Nyabingi, like many other mutual aid initiatives is, in effect, engaging in the recovery process, as one member describes: 'Nyabingi serves people of colour, African and Caribbeans. It's a place where we forge ahead together, working, learning new skills, learning things about ourselves, the way we react with others, sharing happenings, looking out for others' (Anon. quoted in Nyabingi, 2011).

Unfortunately, professionals are often unaware of the significance and potential of mutual aid and can be suspicious of it (Munn-Giddings and McVicar, 2006; Seebohm *et al.*, 2012). This is perhaps because of the individualistic/consumerist emphasis in policies such as personalization. The ethos of mutual aid runs counter to this; reciprocity and experiential knowledge are, by their nature, not things which can be bought and sold. Yet in many ways the current social and policy context favours the development of self-help. On the one hand cuts in services creates a vacuum which mutual aid groups could help to fill. On the other hand, on the surface at least, mutual aid would seem to be in keeping with the government's 'Big Society' policy agenda of citizens taking more control, which *No Health Without Mental Health* (Department of Health, 2011: 3) claims is 'particularly relevant to mental health'. Mutual aid should not be a substitute for statutory provision or a justification for cuts in services. It is, however, something social workers should support.

Group work is one way of doing this, about which Hyde (2013) makes two pertinent points: first, that the 'mutual aid model of group work epitomizes principles of the recovery model in mental health'; and second that, 'Social group work practice has always had a strong self-help focus' (p. 44). Steinberg, writing from the USA, goes further, claiming that mutual aid group work enjoys unique prominence in social work: 'no other helping profession places it as its very epicenter' (2010 quoted in Hyde 2013: 45). Unfortunately, in social work in the UK, group work is not as fashionable as it once was but it is, as Sheldon and Macdonald (2009) dryly point out, 'an efficient use of staff time'. And, to varying extents depending on factors like the composition and purpose of groups, Steinberg's (2014) point that mutual aid is inherent in social work with groups is valid. To realize this potential, social workers must be prepared to share authority and power with group members. Reducing the power differentials can benefit social workers in many ways, one being that in recognizing service users as 'experts by experience' social workers can learn from mutual aid – as a student social worker said of her placement at Nyabingi:

> As a result of the exposure at Nyabingi, I would like to use my practice to dispel the myths surrounding mental ill-health within my own community and use every available avenue to tackle stigma and discrimination of those who suffer mental ill-health. I would recommend the placement highly especially if you don't know much about mental health. Come with an open mind; learn and grow.
>
> (Laura Mburu, 2010 quoted in Nyabingi, 2011: 9)

Poverty, social exclusion and mental distress are closely intertwined: they feed each other, partly because they are all stigmatized. It follows that because mental distress is socially constructed, social workers' skills and expertise can be effective in helping to relieve the damaging effects it has on people lives. This requires a partnership approach, recognizing that service users/survivors do this for themselves. In doing so they can draw on all of Lister's (2004) four types of agency discussed in Chapter 2. Service users and carers do share experiential knowledge of 'getting by', 'getting (back) at' and 'getting out'. Lister's fourth type of agency is 'getting organized'; the service user movement and mutual aid groups are unmistakeably examples of this. Social workers can support service users in exercising all four forms of agency but 'getting organized' can be particularly beneficial for both parties – and fits well with a recovery approach.

Summary of main points

- Mental distress is primarily socially constructed and because it arises out of unequal social conditions is both a cause and consequence of poverty and social exclusion.
- 'Othering', processes of stigma and self-stigma, exacerbates the relationship between mental distress and social inequalities.
- This social construction of mental distress is evident in the sharp inequalities experienced by BME communities which persist partly because of institutionalized racism in mental health services.
- Recovery, as a philosophy developed by the service user movement, is an approach which can assist social workers to work in partnership to support service users and carers.
- Through mutual aid, based on reciprocity and experiential knowledge, service users exercise their agency to overcome the depredations of mental distress.
- Mutual aid is complementary to social work ethics, values and methods and can and should be promoted through, in particular, group work.

Further reading by topic

Social work practice and mental health

Karban, K. (2011) *Social Work and Mental Health*, Cambridge: Polity Press.

Tew, J. (2011) *Social Approaches to Mental Distress*, Basingstoke: Palgrave Macmillan.

Social perspectives on mental health

Friedli, L. (2009) *Mental Health, Resilience and Inequalities*, Copenhagen: World Health Organization.

Rogers, A. and Pilgrim, D. (2010) *A Sociology of Mental Health and Illness*, 4th edn, Maidenhead: Open University Press.

Ethnicity and inequalities in mental health

Fernando, S. (2010) *Mental Health, Race and Culture*, 3rd edn, Basingstoke: Palgrave Macmillan.

Fernando, S. and Keating, F. (2009) *Mental Health in a Multi-ethnic Society: a multidisciplinary handbook*, 2nd edn, London: Routledge.

Mutual aid and the service user movement

Seebohm, P., Henderson, P., Munn-Giddings, C., Thomas, P. and Yasmeen, S. (2005) *Together We will Change: community development, mental health and diversity*, London: Sainsbury Centre for Mental Health.

Steinberg, D.M. (2014) *A Mutual-Aid Model for Social Work with Groups*, 3rd edn, London: Routledge.

Useful websites

Black Mental Health UK: www.blackmentalhealth.org.uk

NSUN (National Service User Network): www.nsun.org.uk

Social Perspectives Network: www.spn.org.uk

8 Making space: tackling poverty and social exclusion

Key messages

- Social work's professional codes of ethics can be usefully supplemented by ethics of care and mutuality. These are 'bottom up' perspectives which recognize the value of caring and mutual aid and thereby offer alternatives to neoliberal individualism.
- In the pressurized practice context of managerialism and high caseloads, social workers can still 'make space' to be better able to support service users struggling against poverty and social exclusion.
- A community orientated approach to practice can enhance social workers' capacity to alleviate poverty and social exclusion, particularly because this approach allows scope to build partnerships with agencies, professionals, service users and communities who are working towards the same ends.

> . . . overwhelmingly it is still the case that people enter social work not to be care managers or rationers of services or dispensers of community punishment but rather to make a positive contribution to the lives of poor and oppressed people.
>
> (Jones *et al.*, 2007: 202)

> Making space, though, isn't it? It's making space, because we don't have time really . . . I want to make sure that if I'm gonna to do the job then I'm gonna do it properly and that I'm actually helping that person: it's not just go and do a review, see that they need the support but then think, 'Well, I haven't got time to do it' . . . You have to make time whether it's liked or not by the people allocating cases . . . I might not get a statistic for it . . . but I know that person's benefited . . .
>
> (Social worker, adult's team)

Having discussed in the preceding chapters how different service user groups are affected by poverty and social exclusion, this chapter looks in more depth at how social workers can tackle poverty and social exclusion. A starting point for this discussion is that, as the quotes above suggest, there is a paradox that permeates social work:

- on the one hand there is 'poverty blindness' in social work (Gill and Jack, 2007);
- on the other hand, many social workers have a passionate commitment to alleviating the effects poverty and social exclusion have on their clients.

There is also managerialism, tightening eligibility criteria and cuts in services. In these circumstances it would be facile to suggest that anti-poverty practice is an easy option for social workers. However, this chapter suggests ways in which tackling poverty and exclusion can be given more prominence in practice by reference to three related aspects of social work:

1 Ethics and values, arguing that social work's professional codes can usefully be complemented by an ethic of care (Barnes, 2007, 2012) and Holman's (1993) mutuality.
2 'Making space' in practice, looking particularly at White's (2009) 'quiet challenges' and Carey and Foster's (2011) 'deviant social work'.
3 Community orientated approaches to practice.

Discussion of anti-poverty and socially inclusive practice should be located in the socio-political context in which social workers operate. To that end the chapter begins by reviewing the tragic death of David Clapson because of what it reveals about the treatment of poor and excluded people in our society.

In July 2013, David Clapson was found dead in his flat. Clapson's unemployment benefits had been sanctioned (that is, stopped or reduced) apparently because he had missed two appointments with an employment advisor. The immediate, medical cause of his death was an acute lack of insulin to treat his diabetes.

> When Gill Thompson, his younger sister discovered his body, she found his electricity had been cut off (meaning that the fridge where he kept his insulin was no longer working). There was very little food left in the flat to eat – six tea bags, an out of date tin of sardines and a can of tomato soup. His pay-as-you-go mobile phone had just 5p credit left on it and he had only £3.44 in his bank account. The autopsy notes reveal that his stomach was empty.
>
> (Gentleman, 2014a)

In protesting against the way he had died, Clapson's sister was anxious that he should not be seen as a 'scrounger'. In fact, he could hardly have been more 'deserving'. Clapson had worked steadily for most of his adult life, including five years in the army and had only stopped work to care for his mother who had dementia. When she died he had tried hard to get back into work. When his sister found Clapson's body there was a pile of CVs nearby. Commenting on Clapson's death a government spokesperson said, 'Decisions on sanctions aren't taken lightly . . .' (quoted in Gentleman, 2014a). Yet in the year Clapson died over 870,000 people had their benefits sanctioned (Gentleman, 2014a).

What do you think? 8.1: The 'deserving' and 'undeserving' poor revisited

Questions for discussion

1 What does David Clapson's case suggest to you about the social circumstances of people who live in such severe poverty? What does it suggest about the policy discourses which determine who gets benefits, which benefits they get and when they are sanctioned?

Comment

David Clapson had had his benefits sanctioned once before, in 2010, and had nearly died then because he had stopped taking his insulin (Lyons, 2014). On that occasion Clapson was rescued by a neighbour. In 2013 he was not so lucky. This is obviously an extreme case, and most people who have their benefits sanctioned do not die as a result. They do, though, often suffer great hardship and in two key ways David Clapson was typical of many socially excluded people:

1 He was vulnerable: he died within weeks of having his benefits stopped and he had a chronic illness which had nearly killed him once before.
2 He was, it appears, very isolated. Even his sister did not know how impoverished he was. A truism of social work is that the more isolated people are, the more vulnerable they are likely to be. Having social networks that can provide reliable support, particularly in crises, makes a huge difference. A common form of social exclusion among service users is that they often do not have such networks.

As with the Work Capability Assessment (discussed in Chapter 3) sanctions on Job Seeker's Allowance (JSA) are punitive and, as a government report has acknowledged, often unfairly hit vulnerable people (Gentleman, 2014a). This is reflected in the growing reliance on food banks. The Trussel Trust, the largest food bank charity, reported a 163 per cent increase in the number of parcels given out in 2013, with welfare reform identified as a major cause (Gentleman, 2014b). This is a measure of the harsh welfare regime that prevails. The government attack on the alleged 'dependency culture' is indeed 'a neo-liberal shock doctrine' (Levitas, 2012a: 322) and vulnerable and excluded people, like David Clapson, are feeling the full force of it. Within this MUD (moral underclass discourse) of social exclusion there is a presumption that people like Clapson are 'undeserving' of help; his benefits were stopped despite, or regardless of, his vulnerability. He was taken to be a 'scrounger' and treated accordingly.

There are people who commit benefit fraud and possibly some who, in David Cameron's phrase, opt to live on benefits as a 'lifestyle choice' (Groves, 2013). Yet the evidence is that non-take up, people not claiming benefits they are entitled to, far outweighs benefit fraud and that government attack on a 'dependency culture' can result in people becoming disconnected from the benefits system and thus more vulnerable to poverty (Finn and Goodship, 2014). This is effectively what happened to David Clapson. He could have appealed against his benefits sanction and may have been eligible for a hardship payment but probably did not know about either (Gentleman, 2014a). Clapson was in a situation that social workers come across frequently: an isolated individual being crushed by structural forces over which they have very little control. A question that then arises is what, in these very hard times, can social workers do about it?

Strier and Binyamin (2010: 1910) argue that 'poverty is simultaneously the expression and the consequence of political, economic, ethnic or gender oppression'. This is a reminder that unequal power relations are central to the experience of both poverty and social exclusion. Strier and Binyamin also warn that social work is implicated in this, citing studies that say that service users often find social services bureaucratic and dehumanizing. It follows from these points that anti-oppressive practice should inform anti-poverty practice. McLaughlin (2005) however, has argued that anti-oppressive practice has been institutionalized and has lost much of its radical content allowing 'the problems of society to be recast as due to the moral failings of individuals who need censure and correction from the anti-oppressive social worker' (p. 300). This analysis can be related to the care versus control continuum in social work. To varying extents depending on the circumstances, social workers can be more or less caring or controlling. Similarly, social workers can decide to be 'personally policing, not politically empowering the disadvantaged' (McLaughlin, 2005: 300). Social workers have choices about how caring or politically empowering their practice is.

Taking the more empowering options can be easier said than done, particularly when practice is so regulated. To practise in an anti-oppressive way, an essential starting point is, as Parrott (2014) says, to be systematic. Parrott describes a four-part process for this:

1 **Assess:** investigate service users' expressed needs, using a strengths perspective.
2 **Plan:** as far as possible in agreement with the service user decide how those needs are to be met in ways which involve the service user drawing on their strengths to play an active part in that.
3 **Intervene:** implement the plan and be clear and in agreement with the service user as to who will do what and in what timescale.
4 **Evaluate:** discuss with the service user what the intervention has achieved and what remains to be achieved and how it can be.

This might sound well and good in abstract but can be far from straightforward in practice. For instance, as was discussed in relation to older people (in Chapter 6) services are often tightly rationed and a social worker might not be able to secure all the resources that he or she thinks a service user requires. There is, of course, a basic principle here: do not promise what you cannot deliver. But there is a wider issue about trying to find ways to support service users and carers more than rationing constraints (eligibility criteria and rapid turnover of cases) might suggest is feasible.

Social care resources are finite but in a situation, as now, where needs are going unmet, social workers can use their discretion and agency to obtain more and better services for their clients than they might otherwise get. Simon Cardy (n.d.) shows this in relation to Section 17 of the Children's Act 1989 under which local authorities' duty to safeguard and promote the welfare of children in need includes financial assistance. With domestic violence, for instance, Women's Aid (2008) argues that Section 17 money can be used for (e.g.):

• cash for new clothes for children;
• cash for travel to get away from a violent man;
• assistance with fitting new locks, getting a telephone or alarm system;
• transport to a refuge.

Cardy's argument is that social workers should be aware of and 'start making demands on these budgets whilst they still exist'. While recognizing the pressure on local authority budgets, Cardy's response to managers is, 'you might control the budget but my job as a social worker is to spend it!'

Ethics and values

Cardy's determination to access resources to alleviate service users' poverty is, of course, a reflection of his ethical commitment. Domain 4 of the Professional Capabilities Framework, 'Rights, justice and economic wellbeing', requires social workers to 'recognise the fundamental principles of human rights and equality . . . ensure these principles underpin their practice . . . [and] understand the effects of oppression, discrimination and poverty' (The College of Social Work, 2012: 2). In the early 1990s, when community care was being rolled out under the NHS and Community Care Act 1990, Bob Holman (1993) criticized social work's professional values as being, 'intensely individualistic', and 'not sufficiently put in a social framework' (p. 51). Nowadays The College of Social Work's (2013) code of ethics enjoins members to 'Serve, and promote the wellbeing of, the whole community' and 'promote social justice'. BASW's (2012b) code of ethics is more explicit, requiring social workers, 'In solidarity with those who are disadvantaged', to strive 'to alleviate poverty and to work with vulnerable and oppressed people in order to promote social inclusion' (p. 5). In this sense the codified ethics and values of the profession have progressed, even as putting them into practice has become harder. Yet, for anti-poverty practice, there are two ways in which these codes can usefully be supplemented – first, with an ethic of care and, second, by mutuality.

The government's attack on the supposed dependency culture emanates from neo-liberal individualism. As Fine and Glendinning (2005: 602) say, autonomy and independence are promoted as the antithesis of dependency and are held up 'as unproblematic and universally desirable goals'. In this view of the world there is a divide between 'those who are needy and dependent on the good offices of others for their capacity to function on a daily basis, and those who are independent, autonomous and have no need for care' (Barnes, 2007: 60). This is a false dichotomy; across the life course people's need for care varies as does their capacity to give it. To give and receive care is integral to the human condition. One problem that follows from the view of dependency as something to be avoided is that it devalues caring and carers. Not only are people who need care socially excluded, so too are their carers:

> The work of care, the washing, dressing, dealing with personal and domestic dirt and damage, is work undertaken primarily by those who are of low social status – women, minority ethnic groups, migrants . . . It is poorly rewarded financially and carried out by those who often have little security or power . . . This both reflects and reinforces the low value accorded to care . . .
>
> (Barnes, 2007: 61)

Neo-liberalism did not create this situation; caring, perceived as women's work, has long been undervalued and poorly rewarded. It has, however, compounded the situation. In this sense, scandals like the abuse of adults with learning disabilities at Winterbourne View, exposed in 2011, are related to the marketization of social care and the consequent casualization of the workforce:

> Social care workers often receive pay below the minimum wage and a significant proportion are operating on 'zero hours contracts'. The 1.4 million care workers in England are unregulated by any professional body and less than 50% have completed a basic NVQ2 level qualification, with 30% apparently not even completing basic induction training.
>
> (Fotaki *et al.*, 2013: 6)

If you wanted to stigmatize caring (and the people who do it), reducing it by privatization, to the status of a commodity to be purchased at the lowest possible price would seem to be an effective way of going about it. If, alternatively, caring and being cared for are activities that we all engage in and which are 'necessary for human well-being, flourishing and indeed survival' (Barnes, 2012: 5) they clearly should be valued. To this end Barnes (2007, 2012) has posited a feminist-inspired ethic of care, based on five moral principles:

- attentiveness: to recognize and be attentive to others;
- responsibility: to take responsibility for action;
- competence: caring should be competently performed;
- responsiveness: consider the position of the care receiver from their perspective;
- trust: is interwoven with power and responsibility and involves 'a willingness to use power in a positive and creative manner' (Barnes, 2007: 63).

These principles are eminently compatible with social work ethics and values and, Barnes argues, are grounded in the experience of people 'whose everyday lives are suffused with . . . giving and receiving care' (p. 71). To that extent, the value of Barnes' ethics of care is that it is based on a 'bottom up' perspective which is emancipatory and sees people, service users and carers as 'experts on the barriers that they face and the means by which they might be overcome' (Dodds and Paskins, 2011: 54). This has much in common with the mutual aid that was discussed in relation to mental distress in Chapter 7. In relation to the principle of attentiveness, for instance, Barnes (2007) cites the example of shared experiences of mental distress in an advocacy group leading to practical supportive action by group members.

If Barnes' ethic of care has its roots in feminism, Holman's (1993) mutuality is developed from Christian socialism. In the early 1990s Holman argued for mutuality as an alternative to the individualism of what was then called New Right (now neo-liberal) ideology. It was this Thatcherite ideology which shaped the NHS and Community Care Act 1990 and the consequent expansion of community care, the legacy of which is evident in, for example, Winterbourne View and the inequalities in services for older people discussed in Chapter 6. For Holman (1993: 57) mutuality is:

- the recognition of mutual obligations towards others;
- stemming from the acceptance of common kinship;
- expressed in joint action;
- towards a more equitable sharing of resources and responsibilities.

Implicit in this is an assumption that cooperation is as inherent to human nature as Barnes argues caring is. Like Barnes, Holman argues that the values he endorses are practical. He acknowledges that mutuality is idealistic but it can, he claims, 'both set out objectives [for a better society] and shape our daily practice' (Holman, 1993: 57). To show this Holman argues four points:

1 Mutuality implies a straightforward application; if we all are of 'common kinship' then we should make judgements about others' social conditions by reference to our own; that is, if we would not want to live with poverty, stigma and exclusion ourselves, neither should we tolerate it for others.
2 Hence 'Mutuality must be based upon right relationships' (p. 59). Anticipating the arguments of *The Spirit Level* (Wilkinson and Pickett, 2009) Holman argues that 'huge differences' in status, power and income are wrong.

3 Far from being anti-individual, mutuality values individuals because we 'have common roots, common needs and common rights' (Holman, 1993: 60).
4 Mutuality will flourish where neo-liberalism is matched by alternatives of greater altruism, equality and cooperation.

Holman's mutuality and Barnes' ethics of care might sound remote from the hard realities of social work practice but they are not. Barnes argues that her theories have developed from her research into the 'lived experience' of older people, people with physical impairments and with mental distress, particularly where they engage in collective action or mutual aid. Holman (1993: 58), who gave up a professorship to work in deprived communities, claims that where he has most found mutuality being practised was:

> ... with the helpers, users and staff at the Southdown Community Centre in Bath. Here I had daily contact with a group of people who shared similar values and objectives, who did not want perks or over-time pay, who were protective of each other, who cared about the interests of others, in whose cause they were prepared to make personal sacrifices.

My argument here is that Holman's or Barnes' ideas complement social work's codes of ethics in ways which can bring them closer to the lives of service users and carers. They can, to paraphrase Barclay (1982), help social workers stand in their clients' shoes. They are thus particularly important when, as now, managerialism works to distance social workers from their clients. These ethics and values can be enriched by what probably compels Simon Cardy to tell his manager that he is going to spend their budget: passion. Theories and ideals best inform practice when they are held with passion. As one social worker explained it to me:

> I feel quite passionate ... having listened to service users' experiences of what it's like and the frustrations they have. You know when you're working with these people every day, I tend to take on board the injustice really and the discrimination ... We are trying to help people to help themselves ... but you could just follow a process and then move on to the next [case] ... But actually for these people to have the confidence to go back and do these things themselves ... there's a lot they could be doing if ... they had that support in just knocking down a few barriers.
>
> (Social worker, adults team)

Making space

Vicky White (2009: 134) argues that since the 1980s social work has experienced major structural and ideological changes which have left many social workers 'disillusioned, disgruntled and under siege'. While social work has been going through these torments, poverty and social exclusion have been increasing both in scale and severity: more people are affected and their poverty is deeper now than it was 30 years ago. In the Introduction to this book I suggested that a starting point of anti-poverty practice is to be critical; Jordan (2012: ix) identifies two key aspects of this:

1 Being aware of what is happening to poor, excluded and marginalized people, and of social work's part in that.
2 Social workers should be active in forging their own destinies, not passively wait for the next round of policy guidance and management instructions.

Managerialism clearly does inhibit anti-poverty practice but need not be a straitjacket. One sign of emerging resistance to neo-liberalism is the growing literature which promotes a revival of radical social work (e.g. Lavalette and Ferguson, 2007; Ferguson and Woodward, 2009). While this has much to offer, Carey and Foster (2011) argue that this perspective has limited purchase among 'frontline' social workers, partly because it has struggled to offer 'tangible, pragmatic or sustainable' (p. 577) methods of meeting the needs of service users and carers. Drawing on the work of White (2009) and Carey and Foster (2011) my aim here is to suggest that there are practical ways social workers can 'make space' to be able to more fully engage with service users' poverty and social exclusion.

Both White (2009) and Carey and Foster (2011) argue that some degree of discretion is inherent in social work practice. In White's analysis there are three general aspects of social work which make it resistant to rigid managerial control:

1 'The difficulty of programming human judgement'; that is, the complexity and variability of service users' needs requires social workers to exercise human judgement – for which machines cannot (as yet) be substituted.
2 From this it follows that social workers have to exercise some discretion; for example about how a service users' needs fit with the FACS eligibility criteria.
3 Because social workers have discretion they also have power, limited though it may be.

These inherent features of social work involve three further factors:

- **Expertise:** in exercising their human judgement social workers draw on a large body of professional knowledge.
- **Indeterminacy:** working in areas of uncertainty in which specialist professional skills are crucial.
- **Invisibility:** practice involves working in situations which do not make close surveillance easy.

The 'McDonaldization' of social work (Dustin, 2007; discussed in Chapter 4) has eroded practitioners' professional autonomy and discretion. White's (2009) argument, however, is that despite this it is in the nature of the job that some discretion will remain and, that being the case, there remain 'nooks and crannies' (p. 143) for resistance to managerialism. This goes back to Jordan's (2012) point cited above about being active: if social workers have power and discretion they can exercise agency. What Carey and Foster (2011) call deviant social work (DSW) is one way of doing this.

From their research, Carey and Foster provide two case studies to explore what they mean by DSW. The first, Pauline (a pseudonym), was an experienced social worker in adults' services who claimed to regularly do 'unauthorized' tasks, primarily as a way of coping with a challenging job in a constraining organizational context. As Pauline explained it:

> It's about tryin' to help the service user or family rather than just tryin' to cover your back all the time or just getting the paperwork done. It's like tryin' to give a purpose to the daily grind of the job . . . Without bending the rules a little it's now almost impossible to help anyone . . . Everyone here knows that you won't get anything from the [funding] panel if you're too honest.
> (Quoted in Carey and Foster, 2011: 585)

Carey and Foster's second case study, Bill, had more than 30 years' experience in statutory social work and had eschewed going in to management. Bill had a 'general distain' for policy initiatives and management cultures such that he 'felt that he had no choice but to evade, disregard and at the very least query aspects of formal procedures and policies' (2011: 587). Bill's rationale for this was about meeting service users' needs:

> What is the point in going out to [the service user's] house and filling out all those forms if there is nothing available [to the user] at the end of all the effort and hard work? . . . I ignore the rules sometimes because the 'system' is unfair.
>
> (Quoted in Carey and Foster, 2011: 588)

Examples of what Bill did when he was 'ignoring the rules' included:

> . . . spending greater time with service users than was permitted, engaging in unspecified 'unprofessional activities', exaggerating needs within assessments or 'panel' applications for support services . . . and confronting middle or senior 'management' about organisational policies within supervision or team meetings.
>
> (Carey and Foster, 2011: 588)

Exaggerating needs was, Carey and Foster (p. 588) say, 'a common reference point' for most of the social workers they interviewed.

Carey and Foster define DSW as 'minor, hidden, subtle, practical, shrewd or moderate acts of resistance, subterfuge, deception or even sabotage that are embroiled in parts of the social work labour process' (p. 578). It is important to emphasize that Carey and Foster were concerned with *positive* deviance which was informed by a 'general sense of empathy . . . towards the apparent plight of service users and informal carers' (p. 590). This approach is, of course, complementary to anti-poverty practice.

White's (2009) 'quiet challenges' are in essence the same type of activities as DSW; she distinguishes two types of resistance to managerialism:

- **Resistance through distance:** this is social workers looking to 'escape or avoid the demands of managerial authority and to distance themselves . . . from the organisation and its prevailing power structure' (pp. 139–40). Bill's behaviour, ignoring the rules and so on, appears to be an exemplar of this.
- **Resistance through persistence:** this requires more involvement in the organization (rather than distancing from it) and involves, for instance, social workers using their expertise to challenge decision-making processes and seeking to hold managers to account. This fits with, for example, what Simon Cardy (n.d.) advocates regarding social workers use of Section 17 funding.

Although the activities they discuss are much the same there is a significant difference between Carey and Foster and White. DSW is posed as an alternative to the radical social work advocated by the Social Work Action Network. White, however, sees quiet challenges as complementary to building a wider movement of resistance to neo-liberalism external to social work practice but which, nonetheless, 'does not have to wait for the fruits of a large-scale transformative radicalism to ripen' (2009: 143).

What do you think? 8.2: 'Just do it', making space in adult services

In the case study below a social worker in adults' services describes how she made space to represent a service user with disabilities at a Work Capability Assessment. Previously she had helped him overcome social isolation by securing a Personal Budget and by getting him a wheelchair.

> [He] got a letter calling him for a WCA . . . [in a town 12 miles from where he lived]. He couldn't go: he couldn't afford to get there. They said they'd give him money for bus fare but he's not near a bus stop . . . So I took him; I picked him up and took him there. And, also, because of his anxiety issues he finds it hard to communicate. So he gets quite anxious and then he forgets about what's wrong with him . . . So I went into the meeting with him . . . And in the meeting he did forget . . . he kept saying about depression and I said, 'Yeah, and you've lost your toe to gangrene and you've had a liver transplant'. And the doctor's like, 'Oh, OK!'. And him, he's like, 'Oh yeah, that as well.'
>
> Usually that's probably not our role, so our managers would go, 'Oh, you've got a review to do . . .'. So I just did it. Otherwise, it's gonna end up: they're gonna make him say he can work and make him sign on, or . . . [stop his disability benefits]. He was getting upset, and he's got no one else to do it, no family, and so I thought the easiest thing to do is, I just put him in the car and took him down there.
>
> To be honest I think that is the kind of thing we should be doing. That is the role of a social worker . . . People [in the team] get frustrated a lot, people go, 'Oh we can't do that, it's not our role to do that any more'. . . So I think, 'Oh just do it!' . . . And a lot of people in the team are probably the same: we just do stuff and it's probably not under our job description any more. But it's what we consider social work to be . . . If you get told off, you get told off!' . . . And our manager's like, she wouldn't say, 'Oh, go and do that' but if you told her you'd done it she'd probably say, 'Oh, that's a good piece of work.' Managers higher up are probably a bit more interested in statistics . . .
>
> But then if you look at it that way, it could have saved us money because in the long run, if he's been told he's got to work and he can't, he's going to get himself more anxious, more upset and that will affect his health. So we could end up having to put more support in. So I could try and wangle it that way.

Questions for discussion

1 In what ways were the social worker's actions 'quiet challenges' to managerialism?
2 How might the social worker's intervention have alleviated poverty and social exclusion?
3 Do you agree that what she did is 'the role of a social worker'? If you were in a similar situation with a service user, would you respond in the same way?

Comment

Taking the service user to the Work Capability Assessment and advocating for him challenged managerialism in that the social worker probably went beyond her formally recognized role. Her challenge was quiet in the sense that she 'just did it'; she did not ask permission to do it or afterwards tell her manager that she had. The outcome of the assessment was that the service user was found to be unfit for work and so was able to continue claiming long-term disability benefits (PIPs). As the social worker suggests, her actions were preventive: if the service user hadn't attended or had been judged suitable for employment, his benefits may well have been sanctioned at some point (when he was unable to work or look for work) and he may well have had a crisis which might have damaged his health and increased his exclusion.

Many social workers would probably agree that what she did was within 'the social work role'. Social work's codes of ethics strongly suggest that the social worker was fulfilling her role. But much depends on the context, on interpretation and on personal values. From a manager's perspective it could be argued, for example, that if social workers did not 'go the extra mile' for service users they could handle more cases and service users would spend less time on waiting lists. Two general points follow from this though:

1 In the end, whether, when and how to engage in 'quiet challenges' is a matter for individual social workers' judgement and conscience.
2 That there is no definitive answer to the question about what the social work role is bears out White's (2009) point about discretion and, therefore, space for quiet challenges being inherent in social work.

Social work and the community

The argument throughout this book is that poverty and social exclusion are best understood as having mainly structural causes. Yet most social work practice, being based on casework methodology, is individualistic. However adept at making space a social worker might be, the contradiction remains: how can individual social workers and service users effectively challenge poverty and social exclusion if the underlying causes are powerful socio-economic processes? There is no easy solution to this dilemma but a starting point is to cultivate more collective ways of working; that is, to develop more of a community approach to practice.

Community social work (CSW) has a history as long as more mainstream social work methods. In the UK it reached its height in the 1980s. The influential Seebohm Report (1968: 147) promoted CSW as: 'a wider conception of social service, directed to the well-being of the whole community and not only of social casualties, and seeing the community it serves as the basis of its authority, resources and effectiveness'. Tellingly, Seebohm added the hope that if this conception of social work was adopted it would sound 'the death-knell of the Poor Law legacy and the socially divisive attitudes and practices which stem from it' (p. 147). Sadly it was not to be, the deserving/undeserving distinction probably has greater prominence now than at any time since the Second

World War. Nonetheless Seebohm's support for CSW was given added impetus by the Barclay Report (1982: xvii) which defined CSW as:

> Formal social work which, starting from problems affecting an individual or group and the responsibilities and resources of social work departments and voluntary organisations, seeks to tap into, support, enable and underpin the local networks of formal and informal relationships which constitutes our basic definition of community.

Any discussion of CSW requires some clarification of what 'community' is understood to be. As Stepney and Popple (2008) say, the term is often used uncritically with, especially, nostalgic visions of a mythical golden past. In social work policy documents and practice guidance there is a tendency to invoke 'community' with little discussion of what it means. For our purposes, Stepney and Popple's (2008: 9) summary is useful. They see:

> ... the definition of community as emanating from the fact that people have something in common, usually in terms of geographical location or shared residence. It is equally possible to consider community in terms of shared elements other than location. For example, links or networks based on religion, ethnicity or occupation.

These two types of community can be summarized as communities of place and of interest. As Stepney and Popple say, the notion that members of a community have something in common is the basis of the 'local networks of formal and informal relationships' referred to by Barclay (above). As was discussed in Chapter 4, there is an argument that communities of place are in decline and giving way to more transient communities of choice. Nonetheless, communities of both place and interest are, as they were in Barclay's day, the basis of the self-help and mutual aid that still provides most social care. That said, although community is usually seen as 'a good thing', it does have its negative side; communities can be racist, sexist and homophobic, exclusionary in any number of ways.

Barclay spurred what Holman (1993) calls the 'summer of CSW' in the 1980s. Typically this involved the decentralization of social services into neighbourhood-based 'patch' teams serving relatively small populations. According to Stepney and Popple (2008) a patch team would probably consist of two or three qualified social workers, community care workers, occupational therapists and local people, paid and voluntary, engaged in various caring and community activity roles. While there was much variation in how the patch system was implemented, its main aspects were: 'a stress on working with people to develop their informal networks; emphasis on early intervention; a concern with preventive action; the desire to utilise and enhance local resources; and ultimately the empowerment of community members for the common good' (Stepney and Popple: 2008: 115).

There is some impressive evidence of the effectiveness of patch-based CSW. Holman (1993) cites research showing that a CSW project on the Canklow estate in Rotherham resulted in a marked reduction in the number of children being taken into care or on supervision orders and a 'drop to almost zero' (p. 75) in the number of children on the child protection register. Holman (1993: 75) ascribes these changes to 'No longer feeling stigmatized and threatened, families came at an early stage of their difficulties [to the CSW team]. The locally run group boosted member's confidence as well as relieving some environmental stress'. At another Yorkshire project similarly impressive results were recorded at the other end of people's lifespans: '. . . working with older people, using local residents as street wardens or homehelps, resulted in a lower proportion entering residential care . . . increased satisfaction with services and improved life expectancy' (Stepney and Popple, 2008: 128).

What do you think? 8.3: CSW and social inclusion

In a critical assessment of the patch system, two points Dominelli (2006) makes are:

1 That it intensified women's exploitation in the gendered inequalities of caring: 'Home helps, street wardens and other ancillary and domestic workers are the backbone of the "patch" system and constitute the bulk of its low paid echelons who are primarily women' (p. 71).
2 That the patch system failed to redistribute 'power and resources in favour of powerless people' (p. 77).

Questions for discussion

1 Given Dominelli's criticisms, how far do you think CSW can go in tackling poverty and social exclusion?
2 What do Dominelli's criticisms suggest about the potential of CSW to change social relations in deprived communities?

Comment

Although there is probably some substance to both points they do seem harsh, particularly given Holman's (1993) point that social workers can alleviate poverty but cannot abolish it. The evidence mentioned above of CSWs effectiveness does suggest that poverty and social exclusion were being ameliorated and it seems unlikely that would have happened if barriers and power imbalances between professionals and service users were not being reduced.

Holman argued passionately for patch-based CSW centred on neighbourhood family centres which would be universal in the sense of being available to everybody in a local community to use. For Holman (1993: 88, 90) such centres should be informed by the values of mutuality discussed earlier. While there is an element of idealism in Holman's argument there is also realism born of long experience of mutual aid projects in deprived communities. He is well aware of their strengths and weaknesses:

> By no means do they attract all residents in happy teamwork . . . participants can argue, blow up, walk out. [Yet] I also know that more frequently they display a readiness to sacrifice themselves, a commitment towards others and an enjoyment of other's company which justifies the description of mutuality.

Not the least advantage of this approach is that it can help realize Seebohm's aim of eradicating the divisive legacy of the Poor Law. Once services become universal, rather than targeted on referrals, the entrenched divide between the 'deserving' and 'undeserving' is removed and stigma begins to be eroded.

Sheldon and Macdonald (2009) assert that much of the literature on community work is 'getting on a bit' which, they point out, might not matter if the social context had remained much the same. To the extent that the CSW literature focuses on the 1980s 'summer' (e.g. Hadley *et al.*, 1987; Holman, 1993) this is a fair criticism – socio-economic conditions have changed markedly, as has policy and practice. As was argued in Chapter 4, since the heyday of the patch system we have had three decades of, more or less, uninterrupted neo-liberalism during which social inequality has become ever more acute. Simultaneously, and for all the rhetoric about choice, the NHS and Community Care Act 1990 initiated a major shift towards managerialism and 'redefined community [social] work away from mobilising people and towards services controlled by local authorities' (Dominelli, 2006: 62). This centralization was compounded by the dominance of crisis-driven, reactive interventions in social work with children and families (discussed in Chapter 5). The summer of CSW was, indeed, brief and since then individualistic methods have been predominant in practice.

Social workers generally have much less scope now to adopt CSW methods than they did 30 years ago. Hence the relevance of 1980s patch-based CSW to practice early in the twenty-first century is not that its methods can be transplanted from the past but, rather, that the general approach remains relevant to the problems poor people face now. This is reflected in the policy context; generally in social policy there is a growing emphasis on prevention which almost demands a community orientation. To complement this there is a new literature emerging which advocates community-oriented approaches to practice (e.g. Pierson 2008, 2010; Stepney and Popple, 2008; Teater and Baldwin, 2012; Featherstone *et al.*, 2014).

There are also signs of 'green shoots of recovery' emerging in practice. The Social Care Institute for Excellence (SCIE) has recently overseen seven adult social care Social Work Practice (SWP) pilots for the Department of Health. These had elements of a community approach, their principles for instance including 'being small, social worker-led and providing strong routes for engagement with people who need or use services' (SCIE, 2013: 1). The SWP pilots were varied in nature but some had a strong CSW orientation. The TOPAZ team in Lambeth, for instance, worked with older people in the borough tackling the contradiction (discussed in Chapter 6) between growing poverty and exclusion, rising need for services and tighter eligibility criteria (The College of Social Work, 2014). TOPAZ has 'three core aims: early intervention, preventive work, and promoting people's independence and wellbeing in the community' (Smith, 2012). As Dee Kemp, the project director claims, 'It's about doing something good for the community, about social justice and grassroots social work' (quoted in Smith, 2012).

Kemp claims TOPAZ is 'what the future of social work may look like' (quoted in Smith, 2012). While social enterprises seem to be expanding in social work, it remains to be seen if a few swallows will make a new summer of CSW. Moreover, for all their positive aspects, there are also trenchant criticisms of the SWP pilots. SWAN (2010) damns them as 'part of a neo-liberal market-testing exercise' and even in a generally very positive report on TOPAZ, Smith (2012) notes that 'No pension, sick pay, maternity leave or job security beyond next year might not sound like ideal terms and conditions'. The SWP pilots may bring new opportunities for more community orientated practice but they also bring the threat of job insecurity and casualization.

Taken together, the policy emphasis on prevention, the new literature on CSW and the SWP pilots might be signs of an emerging new spring, if not yet a summer, of community-oriented social work. If this potential is to be realized we need to be clear about what a CSW approach involves. My earlier point about not transplanting methods from the past notwithstanding, a still useful way of identifying the characteristics of CSW is in the comparison made with traditional social work by Hadley *et al.* (1987). These are set out in Table 8.1. Some of the terminology and related practices mentioned in the table are

Table 8.1 A comparison of traditional and community-orientated approaches to social work

Characteristics of traditional approach	Characteristics of community approach	Changes required for community approach
Reactive	*Preventive/proactive*	
Practitioner reacts to demands for service made when the situation has deteriorated and the user's network can no longer cope.	Practitioner intervenes before a service is demanded and before the situation has deteriorated and the user's network can no longer cope.	1 Reduction of reactive responses, replaced by proactive intervention. 2 Reduction of case-by-case approach based on work of individual professional. 3 Close interaction with the local community.
Services at arm's length	*Services close to the community*	
Professional practice is influenced by departmental programmes, and is completely monopolized by numerous and pressing demands of individual clients.	Professional practice is defined by the living conditions and environmental situation of users and their social surroundings.	1 Variability and flexibility in the method of conceiving, realizing, and evaluating local programmes. 2 Individuals are considered in the round, not compartmentalized by programme. 3 Recognize importance of informal networks. 4 Sharing of professional responsibilities.
Based on professional responsibility	*Based on shared responsibility*	
The practitioner is entirely and exclusively responsible for the solutions to the user's problems.	The practitioner shares responsibility with citizens and/or natural carers.	Practitioners replace, in part, their direct responsibilities by activities supporting others who assume part of the responsibilities.
Centred on the individual client	*Centred on the social network*	
The only target of intervention is the individual client. Evaluation is directed mainly at his/her internal problems and the degree of pathology.	The target of intervention is the social network, including the client's. Evaluation centres on the distribution of responsibility and capacities to adapt.	The practitioner needs to develop skills to evaluate the weight of responsibility experienced by the principal carers, to support them, and to identify and elicit the support of potential users and non-users.

Source: Hadley et al. (1987: 8–9)

clearly dated; for example a social worker would not today discuss a service user in terms of their 'internal problems and the degree of pathology'! Person-centred practice and the strengths perspective seem to have come after Hadley and his colleagues compiled their table. Nonetheless, the utility of the table is twofold:

1 It highlights the differences between traditional and community-orientated practice.
2 By showing the changes required to move from one approach to the other it indicates that this is a *process*, and a matter of *emphasis*. As Sheldon and Macdonald (2009)

suggest, traditional and community approaches are probably best seen as elements of a practice continuum, not mutually exclusive alternatives.

A useful guide to the process of moving from individualistic practice to a more community-orientated approach is Pierson's (2010: 48) 'five building blocks for tackling social exclusion'. As Pierson says, his building blocks are a general guide to promoting the social inclusion of service users which can be used in any area of practice. The building blocks are:

1 Maximizing income and securing basic resources for users and their families.
2 Strengthening social supports and networks.
3 Working in partnership with agencies and local organizations.
4 Creating channels of effective participation for users, local residents and their organizations.
5 Focusing on neighbourhood and community-level practice.

A strength of this model is that it begins where social work practice normally starts, with the individual service user or family, and in steps broadens out to take what amounts to a community-orientated approach. To achieve this, Pierson (2008: 2) argues, 'requires no more than dedication to three broad, flexible themes':

• developing effective relationships with local people;
• utilizing local knowledge;
• viewing social problems holistically.

What do you think? 8.4: Homelessness and sensory impairment

In the case study below a social worker describes how she worked to promote the social inclusion of a family which had suddenly become very excluded:

> I worked with a service user who had visual impairment and significant housing problems who, through no fault of her own, her circumstances changed very, very quickly: she lost her guide dog and she found herself as a single parent so that source of income [her partner's wages] had gone, their home had gone and they found themselves without any support and couldn't get the accommodation they needed.
>
> The partner left and never came back and there were lots of significant debts and ultimately the service user was faced with bailiffs knocking, which was very frightening. So they had to move out very quickly – with the support of [the mother's] family financially but that couldn't be sustained . . . So she found herself at rock bottom . . . at the end of her tether, and didn't know what to do and would have accepted any accommodation – at one point would have been separated from her children.
>
> So in that situation, before we could increase independence, housing was the priority, so working with the district council to try and highlight the issues. This person couldn't live in a hostel because they had four children under the age of 10; had diabetes so needed to store insulin in a fridge but unable to see so wouldn't be suitable for shared

facilities – and yet the option [offered by the local authority] was hostel accommodation or intentionally homeless.

We got the district council to work with us . . . [by] constant calling the housing department, writing letters of support, discussing the case with the GP, flagging up to them, you know: 'Are you aware that this person may be having to share facilities? What will be the impact on their health?' . . . Just bringing other professionals on board to add more weight to this person's case and try to escalate their [housing need] banding higher and higher . . .

In terms of exclusion, lack of awareness of the impact of sight loss in terms of housing . . . you have to go online to bid for houses, for someone who's got no sight, how do you do that? Being offered to go and view a property, a little bit offensive if you think about it!

Trying to navigate your way through the housing system really . . . how hard I found it and I wasn't even the one who needed the home . . . I really found it unbelievable that an agency could leave someone with, it wasn't a choice: 'hostel or nothing'. It wasn't a choice really!

. . . Eventually they were accommodated in a brand new development but, unfortunately, in a very, very isolated location away from services, away from local schools . . . I remember at times there was no mobile signal to be able to contact anybody in an emergency.

So that seemed like a constant battle to try and promote inclusion. They had the accommodation which they were very happy with but, actually, it was completely inappropriate. But through providing assistive technologies so that they could verify the identity of the person at the door before they opened it . . . providing talking kitchen aids so that they can do their own meal preparation without having to depend on a carer; and helping with long cane training and providing a Personal Budget so they could employ someone to clean the home and keep it clutter free so they don't injure themselves, working with health so the diabetes could be controlled . . .

And actually their confidence and resilience developing, so that they've gone on with their lives, and it's been amazing, increased tenfold . . . So resilient how this person actually turned their life around and really we've only played a small part . . .

Questions for discussion

1 Which aspects of this family's social exclusion strike you as most significant?
2 Which of Pierson's five building blocks can you identify being used by the social worker in this case?

Comment

One aspect of this case is the relevance of the social model of disability for understanding social exclusion (as discussed in Chapter 3). The social worker's account highlights how the disabling everyday practice of the local authority housing department exacerbates the service user's impairment (sight loss).

> Most of Pierson's building blocks are addressed in the case study. One area which is not explicitly mentioned is strengthening social networks which might have been done by, for instance, connecting the service user with any local support groups for people with visual impairments. For example, Action for Blind People has local societies. On the other hand, the case study does bring out the significance of the local neighbourhood where the family were rehoused. And, although it is not mentioned, the social worker did work with local agencies to address the problems associated with that.

There are many ways Pierson's (2008) 'three flexible themes' might be pursued but in doing so social workers should choose strategies which are likely to maximize their chances of 'making a difference' to poor people's lives. One such strategy is community needs profiling which Green (2000: 287) argues can give social workers 'the potential to become part of the solution rather than remaining on the margins of the lives of poor people'.

Community profiling (or needs assessment) has developed particularly since the NHS and Community Care Act 1990 required local authorities to assess needs in their areas and plan to meet those needs. As this suggests, profiling is bound up with the notions of needs-led services and evidence-based practice; that is, a profile can provide evidence of needs in a locality on which to base practice responses. Community profiles take many forms and address different needs, including poverty and social exclusion.

Although the terminology is not always adhered to rigorously, Hawtin and Percy-Smith (2007) identify four types of needs assessment which vary in scope and depth according to four criteria, as set out in Table 8.2. The four types of assessment can be seen as a continuum where needs assessment/rapid appraisal is the least comprehensive and has minimal community participation and a community profile is, conversely, the most comprehensive with maximum involvement. Nowadays, it is possible to build up a reasonably accurate picture of a locality from online sources. However, a needs assessment of this kind will lack what are, from a social work perspective, two vital aspects. The first missing ingredient is depth of local knowledge. There are vast amounts of often detailed statistics on socio-economic conditions readily available. However, such statistics will give limited insight into the experience of living in a deprived area. The best way to find out what people feel about their situation, what their priorities are and so on, is to ask them directly. The second missing factor is empowerment, which starts with involvement. If members of a community participate actively in identifying local needs they will probably be more inclined to be active in trying to meet those needs.

Table 8.2 Types of needs assessment

Type	Criteria by which types of needs assessment vary
1 Needs assessment or rapid appraisal	1 The purpose of the exercise
2 Community consultation	2 Who initiates the project
3 Social audit	3 The extent of community involvement
4 Community needs profile	4 The scope of the exercise

Source: adapted from Hawtin and Percy-Smith (2007)

Hawtin and Percy-Smith's (2007: 5) definition of a community needs profile identifies the key elements (in original italics) involved:

A *comprehensive* description of the *needs* of a population that is defined, or defines itself as a *community*, and the *resources* that exist within that community, carried out with the *active involvement of the community* itself, for the purpose of developing an *action plan* or other means of improving the quality of life in the community.

The statistical data referred to earlier is what Green (2000) calls baseline information. This can often be obtained from local authority websites, published as needs assessments or area profiles. A particularly useful source for small areas, such as neighbourhoods or estates, is the Office for National Statistics Neighbourhood Statistics website (http:// neighbourhood.statistics.gov.uk). Using data from such sources a picture of an area can be built up using statistics about, for example:

- the age profile of the population;
- child poverty rates;
- housing tenure;
- household composition.

If, for example, the statistics show that there are, relatively, a large proportion of children and older people in a local population, with high rates of child poverty, a large proportion of social housing and many single-parent and single-person households, this suggests that needs for social care will be high. Such data also begins to give a picture of the multi-dimensional aspects of poverty and social exclusion in that area (Green, 2000). However, on their own the statistics give little insight into the social processes which render people poor and excluded. In the exercise on the 'toxic trio' of domestic violence, substance misuse and mental distress in Chapter 7 (What do you think? 7.3) the social workers' discussion of local sub-cultures shows their local knowledge of the areas in which they work. They will have acquired this knowledge from observing over time what happens in those areas and from talking to people who live and work in them. This is invaluable because:

1 It helps social workers understand service users' poverty and exclusion in its local context.
2 It allows social workers to utilize local resources (formal and informal) in supporting service users.

In these ways a community needs profile can inform ecological practice.

However, given Dustin's (2007) 'McDonaldization of social work', moving to a more community-oriented approach may, as Green (2000) warns, require social workers to make a conceptual leap away from managerialist agendas. It may also require social workers to make space in order to have time and resources to do this. Fortunately the current policy context is amenable to this approach. As well as the general priority now being given to prevention, the government's child poverty strategy recognizes the significance of locality: 'The communities that families live in, and the services and infrastructure that surround them, influence families' prospects of moving into and progressing in work, breaking intergenerational cycles of poverty, and improving children's life chances' (DWP/DfE, 2011: 53). Moreover, the strategy recognizes that 'Some of the most transformative services for vulnerable groups are developed and delivered within local communities themselves and through grassroots-led approaches' (p. 55).

Social workers are not mentioned in the strategy; nonetheless, as Welbourne (2012) suggests, it can potentially give social workers opportunities to develop more community-oriented methods. This is particularly so as local authorities are, under the Child Poverty Act 2010, required to lead partnerships implementing local child poverty strategies which should be informed by needs assessments. The list of agencies to be involved in such partnerships is indicative of the opportunities there can be for social workers to build partnerships. They include, 'Sure Start Children's Centres . . . schools and further education providers . . . [and] local service providers for housing, adult social care, regeneration, transport, and leisure services' (DWP/DfE, 2011: 55). The general point here is that developing partnerships with agencies and professionals working to meet local authorities' statutory obligations can help make space for community-orientated practice. Nurturing mutually beneficial partnerships takes time and commitment but can be done.

Complementary to partnership working, the other side of the coin in a sense, is Pierson's (2010) second building block, 'strengthening social supports and networks'. There are two aspects to this: first, the informal networks of support that people have with family, friends and neighbours and, second, more local voluntary organizations which can provide more formal support. Social capital, relationships of trust and reciprocity can be a critical factor in people's wellbeing but as Jack (2004: 376) points out, 'It is often the groups or individuals who are in the greatest need of additional, more reliable or more satisfying sources of support who are least likely to have access to them'. This is true of service users generally – social isolation erodes wellbeing and compounds disadvantage. In particular, people's ability to cope with crises in their lives partly depends on the extent and quality of the support networks they can call on.

People with low social capital are often hidden from view; the fact that they are isolated can make that isolation harder to spot. This again is an area where local knowledge and being 'tapped into' local networks can make a difference. As well as identifying needs, a key aim of a community profile is to recognize local resources which can help meet those needs. While it appears to be true that social capital tends to be lower in more deprived areas (Jack, 2004) it is also the case that perspectives which pathologize poor people tend to overlook the extent to which they use mutual aid to offset the effects of poverty and exclusion. With some irony, Bob Holman (1993) points out that Easterhouse, a large and very deprived social housing estate in Glasgow, was cited by Charles Murray as an example of a 'feckless' underclass community, yet there are over 300 community groups there: 'tenants' associations, furniture stores, food co-ops, play schemes, welfare rights projects, daycare centres, credit unions, community transport schemes and so on' (p. 87). At the other end of the UK, research in a small but similarly stigmatized London overspill town found some 200 local groups (Harvey and Backwith, 2000). Turning to more informal support, Holland et al. (2011) argue that although networks: '. . . can vary widely in quality and quantity, and are by no means universally available . . . nonetheless family members and friends . . . [provide] informal, material and emotional support for parents, particularly, women living in disadvantaged neighbourhood environments' (p. 410).

Mutual aid, both formally organized and informal has, as Burns and Taylor (1998: 1) argue, 'always been an important way for individuals to cope with immediate needs, with poverty and with social exclusion'.

In the current climate, tackling poverty and social exclusion is not easy. It means going against the stream both of the stigmatizing discourse of the 'dependency culture' and of the managerialism which constrains practice. The ideas set out in this chapter are not offered as a blueprint but as resources which can be drawn on as appropriate to the practice context. Hopefully what all three aspects of the argument – ethics and values, making space and a community approach – point to is the significance of agency. In an era when services are supposed to be user-led, a community approach to practice can assist social workers to build links with and support the many forms of mutual aid which poor and excluded people engage in. Similarly, the extent to which and the way social workers make space to do this will vary but that there is scope to do so is inherent to the profession. Social work's value base impels practitioners to seek to alleviate poverty and social exclusion. Holman's (1993) mutuality and Barnes' (2007) ethics of care enhance that commitment by adding a 'bottom up' perspective.

Summary of main points

- The current discourse of the 'dependency culture' which depicts often vulnerable people as 'undeserving' and thereby legitimizes a punitive benefits regime exacerbates poverty and social exclusion.
- Barnes' (2007, 2012) ethics of care with Holman's (1993) mutuality offer alternative values to neo-liberal individualism. Being informed by the experience of poor and excluded people they offer a 'bottom up' perspective which complements social work's professional ethics and values.
- In the practice context of the McDonaldization of social work (Dustin, 2007), social workers retain, to varying extents, some degree of discretion and power which can be used to make space to more directly address service users' poverty and social exclusion. White's (2009) 'quiet challenges' and Carey and Foster's (2011) DSW are examples of how this can be done.
- As the causes of poverty and social exclusion are mainly structural, traditional individualistic social work methods are limited in how far they can ameliorate it. Accordingly there is a need to move towards more community-orientated approaches to practice. In policy, practice and the academic literature there are signs that opportunities to do this are developing.
- Community needs profiling is one method of adopting a community-orientated approach. Among the advantages of this method are that inherent in it are opportunities to build partnerships with other agencies and professionals, and with service users and community groups.
- Having strong and reliable support networks, or social capital, can increase service users' and carers' resilience. A community-orientated approach can enhance social workers' capacity to make links with the myriad forms of mutual aid which poor people create and which can offer practical and emotional support to their clients.

Further reading by topic

Making space

Carey, M. and Foster, V. (2011) Introducing 'Deviant' Social Work: contextualising the limits of radical social work whilst understanding (fragmented) resistance within the social work labour process, *British Journal of Social Work*, 41.3, 576–593.

White, V. (2009) Quiet Challenges? Professional practice in modernised social work, Ch. 7 in Harris, J. and White, V. (eds) (2009) *Modernising Social Work: critical considerations*, Bristol: Policy Press.

'Bottom up' ethics and values

Barnes, M. (2007) Participation, Citizenship and a Feminist Ethic of Care, Ch. 4 in Balloch, S. and Hill, M. (2007) *Care, Community and Citizenship: research and practice in a changing policy context*, Bristol: Policy Press.
Holman, B. (1993) *A New Deal for Social Welfare*, Oxford: Lion Publishing.

Community-orientated practice

Featherstone, B., White, S. and Morris, K. (2014) *Re-imagining Child Protection: towards humane social work with families*, Bristol: Policy Press.
Stepney, P. and Popple, K. (2008) *Social Work and the Community: a critical context for practice*, Basingstoke: Palgrave Macmillan.
Teater, T. and Baldwin, M. (2012) *Social Work in the Community: making a difference*, Bristol: Policy Press/BASW.

Useful websites

Child Poverty Needs Assessment Toolkit: www.local.gov.uk/web/guest/cyp-improvement-and-support/-/journal_content/56/10180/4063541/ARTICLE
SCIE Social Work Practice pilot sites: www.scie.org.uk/workforce/socialworkpractice

9 Conclusion: love in a cold climate

> You'd have to be on death's door to get an allocated social worker and be put on the [child protection] register.
>
> (Children's social worker)

> It's quite difficult for newly qualified social workers, particularly if they come into statutory from qualifying. They can start to see social work as the process and procedure rather than the actual practice [with service users] . . . Of course you have to do the recording, it's exceptionally important in social work, but the forms and process that the local authority put on you are the policy and guidance. *But your practice is when you are a social worker and that's what you've been trained to do.*
>
> (Social worker, statutory adults' services)

In the introduction to this book it was argued that in the current climate responding to poverty and social exclusion presents particular challenges for social workers for three related reasons:

1 Poverty and social exclusion are getting much worse.
2 Poor people are being denied access to state welfare on an unprecedented scale.
3 Simultaneously the capacity of, especially, statutory social work to respond to that growing poverty and exclusion is much more restricted than it was.

As this book goes to press, a general election is looming; should this bring a change of government this situation might be ameliorated, but it seems unlikely to be fundamentally changed.

In this closing chapter this difficult context is reviewed, drawing on a method used by Steve Cohen (2006) in his analysis of the 'Orwellian world' of immigration and asylum controls. That is to say, Orwell's concept of doublethink is used to draw out parallels between the extreme poverty and social exclusion imposed on asylum seekers and that currently being inflicted on the general population of the UK. The aim is to highlight three points: first, the injustice of what is happening to both groups; second, the importance of social workers viewing social policies critically; and, third, the need to be aware of some of the ethical dilemmas that are accentuated by this context. The final part of this conclusion then reviews the main arguments made in this book as to how social workers can tackle poverty and social exclusion, focusing on:

- a life course perspective;
- the importance of relational social work;

- ecological theory;
- a community orientated approach;
- the moral argument for making space to alleviate poverty and social exclusion.

On the morning of Sunday 7 March 2010 residents of Block 63 of the Red Road estate in Glasgow woke to find the bodies of three asylum seekers on the ground outside the tower block. Next to the bodies was the wreckage of a cupboard thrown, apparently, to break a hole in the protective (anti-suicide) netting through which the three jumped 150 feet to their deaths. Shortly before they died, Serguei Serykh, his wife Tatiana and his stepson Stepan had been told that their application for asylum in the UK had been refused. They had become 'failed asylum seekers'. The consequence of this decision by the UK Border Agency was that financial and housing support was withdrawn (Green and Harvey, 2010; Scott *et al.*, 2010). Not allowed to work and denied access to benefits the Serykh family faced homelessness, destitution and deportation.

Crawley *et al.* (2011: 6) estimate that there are 'hundreds of thousands' of destitute asylum seekers in the UK whose 'overwhelming lack of access to institutional, social and economic resources denies them a sustainable livelihood, and results in a life that is robbed of dignity and unacceptable by human rights standards'. The social exclusion and impoverishment of asylum seekers is more extreme than it is for the indigenous population; yet its severity highlights four aspects which frame the context of social work practice with poor and excluded people:

1 The re-emergence of absolute, subsistence poverty.
2 A resurgence of stigmatization of poor people.
3 Poverty as a deliberate policy outcome.
4 Orwellian 'doublethink' in social policy.

The near-consensus in the 1960s and 1970s that poverty in the UK was relative was a reflection of the almost complete eradication of starvation at a time of rising living standards and universal state welfare. Those days are gone. For example, a Children's Society survey of schools found that in 2012:

- Nearly three quarters (72%) of teachers surveyed have experienced pupils coming into school with no lunch and no means to pay for one
- Nearly half (44%) of those surveyed found that children are often or very often hungry during the school day.

(Rodrigues, 2013: 3)

The explosion in the use of food banks was outlined in the first chapter of this book; the concern here is with why this is happening and its implications for social work. Commenting on the impact of welfare reform and cuts in benefits in particular, MacInnes *et al.* (2013: 9) say:

> The real value of that support, already low (especially for those without dependent children), continues to fall. Restrictions on housing and council tax benefits also mean it has to go further than ever. For some, state support no longer even stops people from going hungry. This is the significance of food banks. It's not so much the number of people having to turn to them (350,000 in 2012/13, even before the deepest of the cuts) as the reasons for the referrals.

Cohen (2006: 25) describes how asylum seekers have been stigmatized; that is, portrayed as folk devils, a threat to social values, 'along with single mothers, paedophiles, drug-takers and welfare cheats'. Similarly, with the onslaught on the dependency culture which is integral to the welfare reform agenda, MacInnes *et al.* (2013: 9) note that for claimants 'the price of state financial support is discipline and demonization'.

There can be a tendency to treat the social policies that cause both the destitution of asylum seekers and growing poverty and exclusion generally as mistakes. For instance, in an otherwise powerful analysis which shows that approximately half of the people using food banks have had their benefits cut, Cooper and Dumpleton (2013: 3) comment that 'the benefit sanctions regime has gone too far'. This seems to misunderstand the aims of policy. The enforced destitution of asylum seekers is not an unintended consequence of well-intentioned policies; rather, in the analysis of Allsopp *et al.* (2014: 35), 'the UK asylum system in and of itself emerges as a poverty producing machine'. Much the same can be said of welfare reform, which is such a major factor in the growth of food poverty.

Cohen (2006) likens the asylum policy regime to the 1834 New Poor Law under which people were deliberately impoverished and stigmatized as a disciplinary measure, to give them a 'stimulus' to take work in the 'dark, satanic mills' of the Industrial Revolution. Today, denial of access to benefits, forced dispersal and the prohibition on working is intended to persuade asylum seekers to return to the countries from which they have fled. Similarly the aim of welfare reform, which could more accurately be called a twenty-first-century New Poor Law, is to 'motivate' people to work in a globalized labour market where low pay and job insecurity is endemic:

- 'In 2012, 4.9 million people were paid below the living wage of £7.45 an hour' (MacInnes *et al.*, 2013: 8).
- Since 2009 the number of people claiming JSA at any one time has fluctuated around 1.5 million. Yet in the two years to 2013 some 4.8 million different people have claimed the benefit (MacInnes *et al.*, 2013).

These two points together are further evidence of people moving in and out of employment but rarely being able to escape the clutches of poverty, as in Shildrick *et al.*'s (2012) 'low-pay, no-pay cycle'. Cohen's (2006: 114) reminder could hardly be more timely, 'Poverty has always been a method for controlling the poor'.

What do you think? 9.1: Family poverty: class and control

Towards the end of their study of poverty, parenting and children's wellbeing Hooper *et al.* (2007: 109) write:

> Parents sometimes think that professionals see as neglect what is really just poverty. Professionals we interviewed were confident (and convincingly so) that they did not, although they were concerned that middle-class neglect was less likely to be recognised than 'the kind of neglect' associated with poverty.
>
> Where resources are scarce and thresholds for intervention high, poverty alone is unlikely to be enough to trigger concern. However in making the distinction between poor families in which children are adequately cared for and those in which they are not, poverty itself often slipped

out of sight in relation to the latter as they focused instead on 'the other things' that made the difference, often parents' priorities, values and attitudes as well as known risk factors (such as drug problems).

Questions for discussion

1 Given what is known about the link between poverty and child maltreatment (see Chapter 5) why do you think that in practice with parents who are struggling there is a tendency for professionals to let poverty 'slip out of sight'?
2 How can social workers guard against the biases described in the extract?

Comment

The tendency to overlook poverty highlights the importance of social workers having a rounded understanding of it. This means going beyond pathological explanations which portray poor people's behaviour as causing their poverty and understanding the impact that poverty and social exclusion can have on people's lives, especially when there is little real prospect of escaping from it. As Hooper et al. (2007: 97) say, 'lack of attention to the impacts of trauma, addiction and lifelong disadvantage . . . may contribute to overemphasising agency at the expense of structural inequality'. This accords with Holman's (1978) explanation (discussed in Chapter 2) of why 'cultures of poverty' can occur in socially excluded families. Another factor can be that, with the urgency to 'make a difference' but with very limited resources, there can be a temptation to address immediately apparent presenting issues rather than underlying structural causes.

To some extent this tendency to pathologize poor people is inherent in what Jones (2002: 17) calls the 'individualism and familialism within social work theory and practice'. If poverty and exclusion are understood as having mainly structural causes it follows that addressing the impact on service users requires a wider approach than social work's traditional individualism. This is part of the rationale for a community-orientated approach. Related to individualism is social control; as is alluded to in the extract, poor working-class families are subjected to much greater surveillance and intervention than middle class ones (see Chapter 5).

Doublethink is a concept first used by George Orwell (1987: 37, 223) in his dystopian novel *Nineteen Eighty-Four* where it explains the capacity of the state to hold contradictory positions and policies and to deny self-evident truths:

> To know and not to know, to be conscious of complete truthfulness while telling carefully constructed lies . . . The power of holding two contradictory beliefs in one's mind simultaneously, and accepting both of them . . . to forget any fact that has become inconvenient . . .

Cohen's (2006) *Deportation is Freedom* uses doublethink to expose the social injustice and hypocrisy of the asylum regime. One example he gives is former Labour Prime Minister Tony Blair's claim in a policy document that 'traditional British tolerance' is under threat from people (asylum seekers) 'abusing our hospitality' (Blair quoted in Cohen, 2006: 20). As Cohen points out, in this view of the world, 'Intolerance (racism) is no longer the product of the racists but of their victims who misuse "our" hospitality simply by their presence here' (p. 20). There is no shortage of research documenting the extreme exclusion and poverty of asylum seekers; for instance a study of failed asylum seekers in 2008 (Taylor 2009) found that:

- 38 per cent had fled their country of origin leaving children behind;
- 54 per cent had been imprisoned and 70 per cent had been tortured.

And that while in the UK:

- their average income was £7.65 per week;
- 72 per cent had slept rough;
- 29 per cent had worked illegally or in 'underground' jobs including prostitution.

Two perhaps obvious points follow from such findings:

1   Only doublethink could allow such impoverishment to be called 'tolerance'.
2   It is surely testament to how real their need for refuge is that so many asylum seekers, 'hundreds of thousands' (Crawley *et al.*, 2011) endure prolonged periods of extreme deprivation rather than return to their country of origin?

Doublethink is also evident in welfare reform. The coalition government's welfare reform strategy asserts that the 'root causes of poverty [are] family breakdown; educational failure; drug and alcohol addiction; severe personal indebtedness; and economic dependency' (Secretary of State for Work and Pensions, 2010: 1). Leaving aside that these are symptoms more than causes, this is as if neo-liberal globalization and the de-industrialization and casualization that accompany it (see Chapter 4) have never happened. Similarly with the rhetoric about the 'culture of dependency' which is contradicted, once again, by authoritative research which finds that 'attempts to portray the workless as a breed apart are quite at odds with the evidence' (MacInnes *et al.*, 2013: 9).

Doublethink and stigmatization come together in the 'Troubled Families' programme. At the time of writing Louise Casey, director general of the Troubled Families programme, has just revealed in a newspaper interview that, on top of the original 120,000, the government has identified a further 400,000 'troubled families'. This revelation came under the headline, 'Rise of the New Underclass costs £30bn' (Hellen, 2014). Levitas (2012b) has made a convincing critique of the dubious evidence base for the original estimates of the Troubled Families programme. Yet, apparently oblivious to this, Casey now claims that this 'underclass' is half a million strong and that 'frankly they cause the most problems and frankly you wouldn't want to live with them' (quoted in Hellen, 2014). Much like the underclass debate of the early 1990s (see Chapter 3) the details of the research that led to this new discovery are sketchy. There is, in Williams' (2014) phrase, 'much more anecdote than evidence'. Unrepresentative horror stories of just how much trouble these families allegedly cause abound; thus far at least, hard data is conspicuous by its absence.

The welfare reform strategy also claims that there will be a 'focus on prevention and early intervention' (Secretary of State for Work and Pensions, 2010: 8). Which seems questionable when, for example, research by Action for Children (2013: 4–5) finds that:

> not only are children facing far greater pressures, but the service infrastructure they depend on is fragmenting. Vital early help is at risk of disappearing . . . [and] With continuing media interest in child protection, local authorities are

placed in an impossible position of meeting devolved responsibilities with ever diminishing resources . . . All the while, the families we work with are at breaking point.

Since the economic collapse of 2008 and the general election of 2010 the landscape of practice with poor and excluded people has shifted dramatically. To the extent that the post-Second World War universal welfare state was concerned with social solidarity and equality, that is no more. One purpose of comparing the social policy regime which governs asylum seekers and that for poverty and exclusion generally is to highlight how harsh the latter has become. As Humphries (2004) has argued, the inhumanity and injustice of the asylum regime presents social workers with sharp ethical dilemmas. In practice, generally, social workers are increasingly caught between the rock of cuts in services and tighter eligibility and the hard place of growing poverty and social exclusion. There is little prospect of that changing in the foreseeable future. The likelihood is that far from being 'eradicated' child poverty will increase, up until 2020 at least (Browne *et al.*, 2013). There is no obvious reason why the problems associated with child poverty should not increase with it. As we have seen the consequences of child poverty include child maltreatment and damage to health and wellbeing across the life course.

In her critique of social work involvement in the asylum regime under the Labour government of 1997 to 2010, Humphries (2004: 95) notes how the policy rhetoric about, for example, choice, citizenship and autonomy coincided with social work values but: '. . . at the same time the government pursues neo-liberal economic and morally repressive policies that systematically degrade public services and punish and exclude those regarded as having been "given a chance" but having "failed"'. With asylum seekers, Humphries (2004: 102) argues, 'Social workers have been drawn in increasingly as part of the surveillance process'. Similarly with austerity under the coalition government, Jordan and Drakeford (2012: 3) argue that 'social work is coming to play a front line role in the authoritarian aspects of the new regime . . .'. But, they add, opportunities are there for the profession to 'recapture its emancipatory traditions'.

What do you think? 9.2: Authoritarian social work?

Humphries (2004: 94) points out that social workers deal with 'the most vulnerable people in society', and with asylum seekers are 'faced with some of the most oppressed people on the planet'. Yet in this work, Humphries argues, social work has been sucked into a role of 'constriction and punishment'. And, she claims, this goes beyond work with asylum seekers: 'there could be no clearer example of the transformation of social work from a concern with welfare to a position of authoritarianism . . . paralleling a more general change . . . towards a culture of blame and enforcement'.

Questions for discussion

1 Drawing on your knowledge and experience of social work, can you think of any examples of policy or practice that support Humphries' criticisms?
2 Given social work's commitments to, for example, social justice and anti-oppressive practice, why do you think social workers might get drawn into the authoritarianism that both Humphries and Jordan and Drakeford (2012) describe?

Comment

There is little doubt that social work practice has become much more constricted than it was 20 or 30 years ago. For example, commenting on a television documentary about child protection social work, Featherstone *et al.* (2014: 106) say they were struck by the 'lack of meaningful, hands-on, practical support offered . . . [and] a seeming preference for telling the parents what they needed to do . . . This seemed a far cry from the kinds of humane compassionate practice that we would consider essential'. On the other hand, in the research for this book, many social workers expressed a strong commitment to alleviating poverty and social exclusion and empathy for people who are excluded. My sample was not representative but it seems likely that the majority of social workers have similar views (see for example Jones, 2002).

Social work is a profession under pressure, both from attacks by politicians and the media and from having relatively fewer resources to meet growing need. In these circumstances it is not surprising that social workers might get drawn into defensive, risk-averse practice, particularly in the statutory sector where managerialism predominates. Moreover Humphries (2004) argues that social work 'is imbued with an individualistic and unpoliticized view of "values"' which renders the profession susceptible to authoritarian pressures.

Social workers are under pressure to 'see, solve and shut' cases which restricts opportunities to build relationships with clients and, thereby, take a holistic view of their situation. For example, a social worker in an older people's team described how demeaning and limited assessments can be:

> It is intimidating . . . you go through the needs of someone and then you get to the part, 'Can we talk about money now?' . . . you have to go through very personal information and, you know, do you really want to tell a stranger that? . . . To tell me their whole daily routine when they've met me for the first time and probably won't see me again, it's just very intimidating, I wouldn't want to be on the other end.

This case management approach could be seen as promoting social exclusion rather than ameliorating it. Whatever methods social workers use to try to alleviate poverty and social exclusion, the starting point is in developing relationships with clients. For instance, in Chapter 8 Pierson's (2010) five building blocks for tackling social exclusion were discussed as a way of moving from an individual focus to a more collective approach. But in different ways each of the five blocks, from income maximization to community-level practice, requires and should be based on relational social work with service users and carers. One experienced social worker presented this to me as non-negotiable:

> The relationship in social work is the most important thing there is . . . I would hope that I would never, ever lose that, because that is what social work is about . . . I don't see how you can get to what it is someone wants to achieve, what the issue is, if you haven't got a relationship with them. Because I certainly wouldn't sit there with someone I didn't have a relationship with . . . and really get to the

root of the issues . . . That's what keeps me passionate about social work, and that's never, *that's never* changed for me.

(Social worker, adults team)

An argument of this book, developed in Chapter 4, is that for understanding how people's lives have been, or are likely to be, affected by poverty and social exclusion a life course perspective is particularly useful. This is because it gives insight into the cumulative impact of disadvantage on a person's life, in part by locating it in its social context. As was suggested with older people, for example, understanding their current situation, particularly from their perspective, requires knowledge of how their previous life history brought them to where they are. It is hard to see how such knowledge and understanding can be gained, other than in the most superficial way, without social workers developing a relationship with their clients.

That can be easier said than done. Yet, as denigrated and restricted as the profession currently is, social workers have status and autonomy which their clients generally do not. There have been high levels of poverty and inequality in the UK since the 1980s. The apparent permanence of this disadvantage might encourage social workers' to lapse into poverty blindness, an acceptance of poverty as an inevitable part of the landscape of practice. This is where Holman's (1993) values of mutuality are relevant, as a reminder that the ravages of poverty and deprivation that are inflicted on, often, the most vulnerable people in society are unacceptable, for us as for them. Values are a spur to action and, as was argued in Chapter 8, because discretion is inherent to social work, opportunities can be found in practice to make space to do more to address poverty and social exclusion.

Complementary to both a life course perspective and a community-orientated approach is ecological theory. Because it involves looking at the interaction of the totality of social relations as they impact on people's lives, an ecological perspective also fits well with a structural analysis of the causes of poverty and exclusion. The tenets of ecological theory were outlined in Chapter 5 in relation to children and families. Jack and Gill (2010a) describe how an ecological perspective can be applied to five levels, or spheres, in assessing the economic or financial aspects of a family's poverty:

- **Household resources:** as well as maximizing income this involves assessing debts and essential expenditure and relating both to any family characteristics which particularly affect household finances; disability for instance incurs additional expense.
- **Wider family resources:** particularly in times of crisis people often rely on their wider family network for financial support. This can be short- or long-term and may affect social/emotional relations between, for example, parents and grandparents.
- **Community resources:** for families living on low incomes the type and availability of resources in the wider community can make a significant difference. In some neighbourhoods there is a relative abundance of credit unions, advice services, child care and other community-run services. In others there are very few, so assessments should take account of this. Social workers will be able to do this more effectively if they have a working knowledge of a family's neigbourhood.
- **Formal institutions:** for this Jack and Gill (2010a) give the example of schools where again there is great variation. Some schools are keenly aware of the ways poverty can affect children's learning and social inclusion and so provide breakfast clubs, subsidies for school uniforms and trips, and other support. Others do little.
- **Wider society:** relative poverty is concerned with people not having the means to participate in normal social life, so cultural factors need to be taken into account.

We have seen, for instance, the importance poor parents can attach to having the latest mobile phone and how for children not being able to join in activities at school can lead to social exclusion.

As well as building up as complete a picture as possible of a family's economic circumstances, the utility of an ecological perspective is that it helps social workers to understand how factors in different spheres can interact in ways which will affect, for good or ill, the people being assessed. An ecological perspective can be applied with all service user groups, not only children and families, and can be applied to different aspects of service users' lives. Much the same approach as that described above in relation to economic/financial factors can be used to understand people's social circumstances, including the extent, nature and quality of their support networks. And, as the example of the cultural importance of mobile phones suggests, economic and cultural factors overlap and interact.

In both theory and practice, there is no clear distinction between relative poverty and social exclusion: both are concerned with people's ability to participate in society. This helps to explain why most of the people social workers support are poor and excluded. For vulnerable people, the availability and reliability of social support networks are major mitigating factors. In turn the social support that service users and carers can draw on partly depends on where they live, the character of their local community. Two points follow from this:

1 Ameliorating poverty and social exclusion is, or should be, integral to social work practice.
2 Social workers' capacity to do this can be enhanced by adopting a community-oriented approach.

As was argued in Chapter 8 there is no blueprint for a community approach and rather than seeing them as opposites it is more useful to think in terms of a continuum with individualistic, casework-based methods at one pole and CSW at the other. Many of the components of a community-oriented approach build on individualistic practice. As the main causes of poverty and exclusion lie in socio-economic conditions and relations, taking a broader approach can give social workers more resources to draw on than might otherwise be available. Foremost among these is mutual aid – the agency of poor and excluded people working collectively to better their conditions of life. As I have tried to show, poor people do this in many ways, formally and informally, to address different needs or aspects of poverty and exclusion.

Mutual aid is complementary to social work in that it builds resilience, it draws on disadvantaged people's strengths and thereby empowers them; that is, they empower themselves. For these reasons it can, as Steinberg (2014) suggests, be seen as being implicit in most social work practice, or at least it has the potential to be. Taking a more community-oriented approach to practice can be a means of realizing that potential.

In advocating a community approach to practice I have sought to follow Teater and Baldwin (2012) in trying to avoid prescribing methods which are not feasible in the current practice context. This is why I have described it as an *approach*, one that can be adopted to varying extents depending on the situation. In statutory settings, especially, social workers will probably have to 'make space' to adopt this more holistic way of working. But quiet challenges (White, 2009) and DSW (Carey and Foster, 2011) are practical options which, in all likelihood, many social workers engage in. Nonetheless, there is an element of idealism in my argument – fully-fledged CSW is far removed from the MacDonaldized version of practice that many social workers are caught up in. To get to that ideal does require, as Teater and Baldwin (2012) say, a paradigm shift. The need to liberate and revive social work is one reason why the profession, and individual social workers, would be better off discarding its attachment to political disengagement. Another reason for social work to be politically engaged is to oppose the crushing poverty that is being imposed on millions of people for the sake of austerity and in the guise of welfare reform.

To paraphrase the Marmot Review Team (2010: 37–8) slightly, poverty and social exclusion are a matter of life and death, of health and sickness, of wellbeing and misery. '[The] case for action is principally a moral one. The fact that people on low incomes lose 17 years of disability free life because they live in worse conditions than people on high incomes is reason enough to act.'

Appendix

Fair Access to Care Services (FACS) bandings and eligibility criteria for individuals

Critical – when:

- life is, or will be, threatened; and/or
- significant health problems have developed or will develop; and/or
- there is, or will be, little or no choice and control over vital aspects of the immediate environment; and/or
- serious abuse or neglect has occurred or will occur; and/or
- there is, or will be, an inability to carry out vital personal care or domestic routines; and/or
- vital involvement in work, education or learning cannot or will not be sustained; and/or
- vital social support systems and relationships cannot or will not be sustained; and/or
- vital family and other social roles and responsibilities cannot or will not be undertaken.

Substantial – when:

- there is, or will be, only partial choice and control over the immediate environment; and/or
- abuse or neglect has occurred or will occur; and/or
- there is, or will be, an inability to carry out the majority of personal care or domestic routines; and/or
- involvement in many aspects of work, education or learning cannot or will not be sustained; and/or
- the majority of social support systems and relationships cannot or will not be sustained; and/or
- the majority of family and other social roles and responsibilities cannot or will not be undertaken.

Moderate – when:

- there is, or will be, an inability to carry out several personal care or domestic routines; and/or
- involvement in several aspects of work, education or learning cannot or will not be sustained; and/or
- several social support systems and relationships cannot or will not be sustained; and/or
- several family and other social roles and responsibilities cannot or will not be undertaken.

Low – when:

- there is, or will be, an inability to carry out one or two personal care or domestic routines; and/or
- involvement in one or two aspects of work, education or learning cannot or will not be sustained; and/or
- one or two social support systems and relationships cannot or will not be sustained; and/or
- one or two family and other social roles and responsibilities cannot or will not be undertaken.

Source: Department of Health (2010: 21)

Note: at the time of writing the FACS criteria are due to be replaced by a National Eligibility Threshold under the Care Act 2014.

References

Action for Children (2012) *The Red Book 2012: the annual review of the impact of spending decisions on vulnerable children and families*, Watford: Action for Children.

Action for Children (2013) *The Red Book 2013: children under pressure*, Watford: Action for Children.

Age UK (2011) *A Snapshot of Ageism in the UK and across Europe*, London: Age UK.

Age UK (2012) *Agenda for Later Life 2012: policy priorities for active ageing*, London: Age UK.

Alcock, P. (2006) *Understanding Poverty*, 3rd edn, Basingstoke: Palgrave Macmillan.

Aldridge, H., Kenway, P., MacInnes, T. and Parekh, A. (2012) *Monitoring Poverty and Social Exclusion 2012*, York: Joseph Rowntree Foundation.

Allsopp, J., Sigona, N. and Phillimore, J. (2014) *Poverty Among Refugees and Asylum Seekers in the UK: an evidence and policy review*, Birmingham: Institute for Research into Superdiversity, University of Birmingham.

Amas, N. (2008) *Housing, New Migration and Community Relations: a review of the evidence base*, London: Information Centre about Asylum and Refugees.

Arai, L. (2009) What a Difference a Decade Makes: rethinking teenage pregnancy as a problem, *Social Policy and Society*, 8.2, 171–83.

Bacino, L. (2014) Shock Figures Show Extent of Self-harm in English Teenagers, *The Guardian*, 21 May, available at: www.theguardian.com/society/2014/may/21/shock-figures-self-harm-england-teenagers, accessed 21 June 2014.

Bambra, C. (2008) Incapacity Benefit Reform and the Politics of Ill Health, *British Medical Journal*, 337, a1452.

Barclay, P.M. (1982) *Social Workers: their role and tasks* (The Barclay Report), London: Bedford Square Press.

Barnard, H. and Turner, C. (2011) *Poverty and Ethnicity: a review of evidence*, York: Joseph Rowntree Foundation.

Barnardo's (2011) *Tackling Child Poverty and Improving Life Chances: consulting on a new approach [response]*, London: Barnardo's.

Barnes, C. (2004) *Independent Living, Politics and Implications*, Leeds: Centre for Disability Studies, available at: www.leeds.ac.uk/disability-studies/archiveuk/Barnes/Jane's%20paper.pdf.

Barnes, J. (2007) *Down Our Way: the relevance of neighbourhoods for parenting and child development*, Chichester: John Wiley & Sons.

Barnes, M. (2007) Participation, Citizenship and a Feminist Ethic of Care, Ch. 4 in Balloch, S. and Hill, M. (2007) *Care, Community and Citizenship: research and practice in a changing policy context*, Bristol: Policy Press.

Barnes, M. (2012) *Care in Everyday Life: an ethic of care in practice*, Bristol: Policy Press.

Barr, B., Taylor-Robinson, D., Scott-Samuel, A., McKee, M. and Stuckler, D. (2012) Suicides Associated with the 2008–10 Economic Recession in England: time trend analysis, *British Medical Journal*, 345 (Aug 13, 2).

Bartley, M. (ed.) (2012) *Life Gets Under Your Skin*, London: UCL Research Department of Epidemiology and Public Health.

Bartley, M., Blane, D. and Montgomery, S. (1997) Health and the Life Course: why safety nets matter, *British Medical Journal*, 314, 1194–6.

BASW (2012a) *The State of Social Work 2012*, Birmingham: BASW.

BASW (2012b) *The Code of Ethics for Social Work: statement of principles*, Birmingham: BASW.

Becker, S. (1997) *Responding to Poverty: the politics of cash and care*, London: Longman.

Beider, H. and Netto, G. (2012), Minority Ethnic Communities and Housing: access, experiences and participation, Ch. 5 in Craig, G. Atkin, K. Chattoo, S. and Flynn, R. (eds) *Understanding 'Race' and Ethnicity: theory, history, policy, practice*, Bristol: Policy Press.

Bell, K. (2013) Poverty, Social Security and Stigma, *Poverty*, spring, 114, 10–13.

Belsky, J. and Melhuish, E. (2007) Impact of Sure Start Local Programmes on Children and Families, Ch. 8 in Belsky, J., Barnes, J. and Melhuish, E. (eds) *The National Evaluation of Sure Start: does area-based early intervention work?* Bristol: Policy Press.

Beresford, P. (1996) Poverty and Disabled People: challenging dominant debates and policies, *Disability & Society*, 11.4, 553–68.

Beresford, P. (2009) *Whose Personalisation?* Think Pieces No. 47, London: Compass.

Beresford, P., Green, D., Lister, R. and Woodard, K. (1999) *Poverty First Hand: poor people speak for themselves*, London: CPAG.

Beresford, P., Nettle, M. and Perring, R. (2010) *Towards a Social Model of Madness and Distress? Exploring what service users say*, York: Joseph Rowntree Foundation.

Birrell, I. (2011) The demonisation of the disabled is a chilling sign of the times, *The Observer*, available at: http://www.theguardian.com/commentisfree/2011/dec/04/ian-birrell-prejudice-against-disabled.

Blair, T. (2010) *A Journey*, London: Hutchinson.

Bradshaw, J. (2011a) Poverty, Ch. 5 in Walker, A., Sinfield, A. and Walker, C. (eds) *Fighting Poverty, Inequality and Injustice: a manifesto inspired by Peter Townsend*, Bristol: Policy Press.

Bradshaw, J. (2011b) Child Poverty and Deprivation, Ch. 3 in Bradshaw, J. (ed.) *The Well-being of Children in the UK*, Bristol: Policy Press.

Bradshaw, J. and PSE team (2013) *Consultation on Child Poverty Measurement*, PSE Policy Response Working Paper, No. 8, available at: www.poverty.ac.uk/report-child-poverty-government-policy-editors-pick/pse-team-slam-government-consultation-child.

Brandon, M., Bailey, S., Belderson, P., Gardner, R., Sidebotham, P., Dodsworth, J., Warren, C. and Black, J. (2009) *Understanding Serious Case Reviews and their Impact: a biennial analysis of serious case reviews 2005–07*, London: Department for Children, Schools and Families.

Brandon, M., Bailey, S. and Belderson, P. (2010) *Building on the Learning from Serious Case Reviews: a two-year analysis of child protection database notifications 2007–2009*, London: Department for Education.

Brawn, E., Bush, M., Hawkings, C. and Trotter, R. (2013) *The Other Care Crisis: making social care funding work for disabled adults in England*, London: Scope, Mencap, National Autistic Society, Sense, Leonard Cheshire Disability.

Brindle, D. (2012) Graph of Doom: a bleak future for social care services, *The Guardian*, 15 May, available at: www.theguardian.com/society/2012/may/15/graph-doom-social-care-services-barnet, accessed 11 April 2013.

Brown, T. (2014) I'm Coming Out, *Scilogs* (blog), available at: www.scilogs.com/epilogue/im-coming-out/, accessed 28 March 2014.

Browne, J., Hood, A. and Joyce, R. (2013) *Child and Working-Age Poverty in Northern Ireland from 2010 to 2020*, London: Institute for Fiscal Studies.

Buchanan, A. (2007) Including the Socially Excluded: the impact of government policy on vulnerable families and children in need, *British Journal of Social Work*, 37, 187–207.

Burchardt, T. (2003) *Being and Becoming: social exclusion and the onset of disability*, CASE Report 21, London: Centre for Analysis of Social Exclusion, London School of Economics.

Burchardt, T. (2004) Capabilities and Disability: the capabilities framework and the social model of disability, *Disability & Society*, 19.7, 735–51.

Burns, D. and Taylor, M. (1998) *Mutual Aid and Self-Help: coping strategies for excluded communities*, Bristol: Policy Press.

Byrne, D. (2005) *Social Exclusion*, 2nd edn, Maidenhead: Open University Press.

Bywaters, P. (2007) Understanding the Life Course, Ch. 13 in Lymbery, M. and Postle, K. (2007) *Social Work: a companion to learning*, London: Sage.

Bywaters, P. (2009) Tackling Inequalities in Health: a global challenge for social work, *British Journal of Social Work*, 39.2, 353–67.

CAADA (Co-ordinated Action Against Domestic Abuse) (2014) *In Plain Sight: the evidence from children exposed to domestic abuse*, Bristol: CAADA.

Cabinet Office (2010) *State of the Nation Report: poverty, worklessness and welfare dependency in the UK*, London: Cabinet Office.

Campbell, J. and Davidson, G. (2012) *Post-qualifying Mental Health Social Work Practice*, London: Sage.

Cardy, S. (n.d.) How should social workers support children and families facing destitution and cuts to their benefits? *Social Work Action Network*, available at: www.socialworkfuture.org/articles-and-analysis/articles/306-how-should-social-workers-support-children-in-poverty, accessed 23 April 2013.

Carers UK (2011) *The Cost of Caring: how money worries are pushing carers to breaking point*, London: Carers UK.

Carey, M. and Foster, V. (2011) Introducing 'Deviant' Social Work: contextualising the limits of radical social work whilst understanding (fragmented) resistance within the social work labour process, *British Journal of Social Work*, 41.3, 576–93.

Carr, S. (2003) Lesbian and Gay Perspectives on Mental Distress, in Social Perspectives Network (2003) *Start Making Sense . . . developing social models to understand and work with mental distress*, SPN Paper 3, London: Social Perspectives Network.

Catney, G. (2013) *Has Neighbourhood Ethnic Segregation Decreased?*, Manchester: Centre on Dynamics of Ethnicity.

Cawson, P. (2002) *Child Maltreatment in the Family: the experience of a national sample of young people*, London: NSPCC.

Centre for Social Justice (2006) *Breakdown Britain: interim report on the state of the nation*, London: Centre for Social Justice.

Centre for Social Justice (2010) *The Forgotten Age: understanding poverty and social exclusion later in life*, London: Centre for Social Justice.

Centre for Social Justice (2011) *Mental Health: poverty, ethnicity and family breakdown*, London: Centre for Social Justice.

Centre for Social Justice (2012) *Transforming Care for the Poorest Older People: a CSJ report ahead of the government's White Paper on social care*, London: Centre for Social Justice.

Chand, A. (2008) 'Every Child Matters?' A critical review of child welfare reforms in the context of minority ethnic children and families, *Child Abuse Review*, 17.1, 6–22.

Channel 4 (2013) *Dispatches: rich and on benefits*, broadcast 18 March 2013, available at: www.channel4.com/programmes/dispatches/4od#3534011, accessed 3 May 2014.

Chartered Institute of Public Finance and Accountancy (CIPFA) (2011) *Smart Cuts? Public spending on children's social care*, London: National Society for the Prevention of Cruelty to Children (NSPCC).

Chief Secretary to the Treasury (2003) *Every Child Matters*, Cm 5860, London: Stationery Office.

Children's Society (2012) *Our Response to the Riots Communities and Victims Panel Report*, press release 28 March, available at: www.childrenssociety.org.uk/news-views/press-release/our-response-riots-communities-and-victims-panel-report, accessed 5 January 2013.

Citizens Advice Bureau (2013) Citizens Advice reports 'Alarming' 78% Rise in Foodbanks Enquiries, press release, 19 August, available at: www.citizensadvice.org.uk/press_office20130819.

Coffield, F., Robinson, P. and Sarsby, J. (1980) *A Cycle of Deprivation? A case study of four families*, London: Heinemann Educational Books.

Cohen, S. (2006) *Deportation is Freedom: the Orwellian world of immigration controls*, London: Jessica Kingsley.

Coldham, T. (2010) Foreword, in Beresford, P., Nettle, M. and Perring, R., *Towards a social Model of Madness and Distress? Exploring what service users say*, York: Joseph Rowntree Foundation.

Cooper, N. and Dumpleton, S. (2013) *Walking the Breadline: the scandal of food poverty in 21st century Britain*, London: Church Action on Poverty/Oxfam.

Coppock, V. and Dunn, B. (2010) *Understanding Social Work Practice in Mental Health*, London: Sage.

Coren, E., Iredale, W., Bywaters, P., Rutter, D. and Robinson, J. (2010) *The Contribution of Social Work and Social Care to the Reduction of Health Inequalities: four case studies*, Research Briefing 33, London: SCIE.

Corker, E., Hamilton, S., Henderson, C., Weeks, C., Pinfold, V., Rose, D., Williams, P., Flach, C., Gill, V., Lewis-Holmes, E. and Thornicroft, G. (2013) Experiences of Discrimination Among People Using Mental Health Services in England 2008–2011, *British Journal of Psychiatry*, 202: s58–63.

Corrigan, P. and Watson, A. (2002) The Paradox of Self-Stigma and Mental Illness, *Clinical Psychology: Science and Practice*, 9.1, 35–53.

Craig, G. (2002) Poverty, Social Work and Social Justice, *British Journal of Social Work* 32.6, 669–82.

Craig, G. (2005) Poverty among black and minority ethnic children, Ch. 5 in Preston, G. (ed.) *At Greatest Risk: the children most likely to be poor*, 65–78, London: CPAG.

Crawley, H., Hemmings, J. and Price, N. (2011) *Coping with Destitution: survival and livelihood strategies of refused asylum seekers living in the UK*, London: Oxfam.

Cribb, J., Joyce, R. and Phillips, D. (2012) *Living Standards, Poverty and Inequality in the UK: 2012*, London: Institute for Studies.

CSIP, RCPsych and SCIE (2007) *A Common Purpose: recovery in future mental health services*, London: Care Services Improvement Partnership (CSIP), Royal College of Psychiatrists (RCPsych) and Social Care Institute for Excellence (SCIE).

D'Cruz, H., Gillingham, P. and Melendez, S. (2007) Reflexivity, its Meanings and Relevance for Social Work: a critical review of the literature, *British Journal of Social Work*, 37, 73–90.

Demos (n.d.) *Poverty in Perspective: working-age childless households*, London: Demos, available at: www.demos.co.uk/blog/workingagepoverty, accessed 30 August 2014.

Dennison, C. (2004) *Teenage Pregnancy: an overview of the research evidence*, London: Health Development Agency.

Department for Communities and Local Government (2011) *The English Indices of Deprivation 2010*, London: DCLG.

Department for Education and Skills (2004) *Every Child Matters: change for children*, London: Department for Education and Skills.

Department of Health (2008) *Health Inequalities: progress and next steps*, London: Department of Health.

Department of Health (2010) *Prioritising Need in the Context of Putting People First: a whole system approach to eligibility for social care – guidance on eligibility criteria for adult social care*, London: The Stationery Office.

Department of Health (2011) *No Health Without Mental Health: a cross-government mental health outcomes strategy for people of all ages*, London: Department of Health.

Dermott (2012) 'Poverty' Versus 'Parenting': an emergent dichotomy, *Studies in the Maternal*, 4.2, 1–13.

Disability Alliance (2010) *The Disability Manifesto: tackling disability poverty*, revised edn, London: Disability Alliance.

Dodds, A. and Paskins, D. (2011) Top-down or Bottom-up: the real choice for public services? *Journal of Poverty and Social Justice*, 19.1, 51–61.

Dolan, A. and Bentley, P. (2013) Vile Product of Welfare UK, *Daily Mail*, 3 April, 1.

Dominelli, L. (2006) *Women and Community Action*, Bristol: Policy Press.

Dominelli, L. (2010) Globalization, Contemporary Challenges and Social Work Practice, *International Social Work*, 53.5, 599–612.

Dorling, D. (2011) *So You Think you Know About Britain*? London: Constable & Robinson.

Dorling, D. and Shaw, M. (2000) Life Chances and Lifestyles, Ch. 12 in, Gardiner, V. and Matthews, M. (eds) *The Changing Geography of the UK*, 3rd edn, London: Routledge.

Drakeford, M. and Gregory, L. (2008) Anti-poverty Practice and the Changing World of Credit Unions: new tools for social workers, *Practice*, 20.3, 141–50.

Duncan, S., Edwards, R. and Song, M. (1999) Social Threat or Social Problem? Media representations of lone mothers and policy implications, Ch. 15 in Franklin, B. (ed.) *Social Policy, the Media and Misrepresentation*, London: Routledge.

Duncan Smith, I. (2010) Foreword to Secretary of State for Work and Pensions *21st Century Welfare*, Cm 7913, London: Stationery Office.

Duncan Smith, I. (2012) Foreword to Secretary of State for Work and Pensions *Measuring Child Poverty: a consultation on better measures of child poverty*, Cm 8483, London: Stationery Office.

Dunning, J. (2010) Count Me In: racial inequalities in mental health services, *Community Care*, available at: www.communitycare.co.uk/2010/02/19/count-me-in-racial-inequalities-in-mental-health-services/#.U2DPx1eGrzK.

Dustin, D. (2007) *The McDonaldization of Social Work*, Farnham: Ashgate.

DWP/DfE (2011) *A New Approach to Child Poverty: tackling the causes of disadvantage and transforming families' lives*, Cm 8061, London, Stationery Office.

Dyson, C. (2008) *Poverty and Child Maltreatment: child protection research briefing*, London: NSPCC.

Eisenstadt, N. (2011) *Providing a Sure Start: how government discovered early childhood*, Bristol: Policy Press.

Emejulu, A. (2008) The Intersection of Ethnicity, Poverty and Wealth, Ch. 8 in Ridge, T. and Wright, S. (eds) *Understanding Inequality, Poverty and Wealth*, Bristol: Policy Press.

Equal Opportunities Commission (EOC) (2007) *Moving On Up? The way forward: report of the EOC's investigation into Bangladeshi, Pakistani and Black Caribbean women and work*, Manchester: Equal Opportunities Commission.

Falkingham, J., Evandrou, M., McGowan, T., Bell, D. and Bowes, A. (2010) *Demographic Issues, Projections and Trends: older people with high support needs in the UK*, York: Joseph Rowntree Foundation.

Featherstone, B., Morris, K. and White, S. (2013) A Marriage Made in Hell: early intervention meets child protection, *British Journal of Social Work*, 44.7, 1735–49.

Featherstone, B., White, S. and Morris, K. (2014) *Re-imagining Child Protection: towards humane social work with families*, Bristol: Policy Press.

Fenton, A., Tyler, P., Markkanen, S., Clarke, A. and Whitehead, C. (2010) *Why Do Neighbourhoods Stay Poor? Deprivation, place and people in Birmingham*, London: Barrow Cadbury Trust.

Ferguson, I. and Woodward, R. (2009) *Radical Social Work in Practice: making a difference*, Bristol: Policy Press

Fernando, S. (2010) *Mental Health, Race and Culture*, 3rd edn, Basingstoke: Palgrave Macmillan.

Ferragina, E., Tomlinson, M. and Walker, R. (2013) *Poverty, Participation and Choice: the legacy of Peter Townsend*, York: Joseph Rowntree Foundation.

Field, F. (1989) *Losing Out: the emergence of Britain's underclass*, London: Blackwell.

Field, F. (2010) *The Foundation Years: preventing poor children becoming poor adults*, London: Cabinet Office.

Fine, M. and Glendinning, C. (2005) Dependence, Independence or Inter-dependence? Revisiting the concepts of 'care' and 'dependency', *Ageing & Society*, 25, 601–21.

Finn, D. and Goodship, J. (2014) *Take-up of Benefits and Poverty: an evidence and policy review*, London: Centre for Economic and Social Inclusion.

Finney, N. and Simpson, L. (2009) *'Sleepwalking to Segregation'? Challenging myths about race and immigration*, Bristol: Policy Press.

Foster, L. (2011) Older People, Pensions and Poverty: an issue for social workers? *International Social Work*, 54.3, 344–60.

Fotaki, M., Ruane, S. and Leys, C. (2013) *The Future of the NHS? Lessons from the market in social care in England*, London: Centre for Health and the Public Interest.

Friedli, L. (2009) *Mental Health, Resilience and Inequalities*, Copenhagen: World Health Organization.

Garnham, A. (2013) The Politics of the Child Poverty Measurement Consultation, *Children and Young People Now*, 6 February.

Garrett, P.M. (2009) *'Transforming' Children's Services? Social work, neoliberalism and the 'modern' world*, Maidenhead: Open University Press.

Garthwaite, K. (2010) Poor Women in Rich Countries: the feminization of poverty over the life course (review), *Times Higher Education Supplement*, available at: www.timeshighereducation.co.uk/ books/poor-women-in-rich-countries-the-feminization-of-poverty-over-the-life-course/411292.article, accessed 20 August 2013.

Gentleman, A. (2010) Is Britain Broken? *The Guardian*, 31 March, available at: www.guardian.co.uk/ society/2010/mar/31/is-britain-broken, accessed 20 August 2013.

Gentleman, A. (2014a) 'No one should die penniless and alone': the victims of Britain's harsh welfare sanctions, *The Guardian*, 3 August, available at: www.theguardian.com/society/2014/aug/03/victims-britains-harsh-welfare-sanctions, accessed 8 August 2014.

Gentleman, A. (2014b) Food Bank Britain: can MPs agree on the causes of poverty in the UK? *The Guardian*, 4 Jul, available at: www.theguardian.com/society/2014/aug/03/victims-britains-harsh-welfare-sanctions, accessed 8 August 2014.

Ghate, D. and Hazel, N. (2002) *Parenting in Poor Environments: stress, support and coping*, London: Jessica Kingsley.

Gill, O. and Jack, G. (2007) *The Child and Family in Context: developing ecological practice in disadvantaged communities*, Lyme Regis: Russell House Publishing.

Glass, N. (1999) Sure Start: the development of an early intervention programme for young children in the United Kingdom, *Children and Society*, 13.4, 257–64.

Glass, N. (2005) Surely some mistake? *The Guardian*, 5 January, available at: www.guardian.co.uk/ society/2005/jan/05/guardiansocietysupplement.childrensservices.

Gordon, D. and Pantazis, C. (1997) Measuring Poverty: breadline Britain in the 1990s, Ch. 1 in Gordon, D. and Pantazis, C. (eds) *Breadline Britain in the 1990s*, Aldershot: Ashgate.

Gould, N. (2010) *Mental Health Social Work in Context*, Abingdon: Routledge.

Green, C. and Harvey, K. (2010) The Estate where Asylum Seekers Abandon Hope, *The Independent*, 9 March, available at: www.independent.co.uk/news/uk/home-news/the-estate-where-asylum-seekers-abandon-hope-1918347.html, accessed 18 June 2010.

Green, H., McGinnity, A., Meltzer, H., Ford, T. and Goodman, R. (2005) *Mental Health of Children and Young People in Great Britain, 2004*, Basingstoke: Palgrave Macmillan.

Green, R. (2000) Applying a Community Needs Profiling Approach to Tackling Service User Poverty, *British Journal of Social Work*, 30.3, 287–303.

Gregg, P. (2008) Childhood Poverty and Life Chances, Ch. 8 in Strelitz, J. and Lister, R. (eds) *Why Money Matters: family income, poverty and children's lives*, London: Save the Children.

Groves, J. (2013) Osborne was right about Philpott, says Cameron, as storm rages on over benefits, *Mail Online*, 6 April, available at: www.dailymail.co.uk/news/article-2304804/Mick-Philpott-benefits-culture-David-Cameron-backs-George-Osborne-saying-arson-case-raises-questions-welfare-lifestyle-choice.html#ixzz2bxI024Bv.

Gupta, A. and McNeill-Mckinnell, M. (2009) The Wider Family and Community, Ch. 3 in Cleaver, H., Cawson, P., Gorin, S. and Walker, S. (eds) *Safeguarding Children: a shared responsibility*, Chichester: Wiley-Blackwell.

Hadley, R., Cooper, M., Dale, P. and Stacy, G. (1987) *A Community Social Worker's Handbook*, London: Tavistock Publications.

Hannen, J. (n.d.) The 'Graph of Doom' and the Changing Role for Local Government, *Greater Manchester Centre for Voluntary Organisation*, available at: www.gmcvo.org.uk/graph-doom-and-changing-role-local-government, accessed 11 April 2013.

Harris, J. (2009) 'Social Evils' and 'Social Problems' in Britain Since 1904, Ch. 2 in Utting, D. (ed.) *Contemporary Social Evils*, Bristol: Policy Press/Joseph Rowntree Foundation.

Harrison, M. with Phillips, D. (2003) *Housing and Black and Minority Ethnic Communities: review of the evidence base*, London: Office of the Deputy Prime Minister.

Harvey, D. (2005) *A Brief History of Neoliberalism*, Oxford: Oxford University Press.

Harvey, L. and Backwith, D. (2000) From Poverty to Social Exclusion? The legacy of London overspill in Haverhill, Ch. 10 in Bradshaw, J. and Sainsbury, R. (eds) *Researching Poverty*, Aldershot: Ashgate.

Hawtin, M. and Percy-Smith, J. (2007) *Community Profiling: a practical guide*, 2nd edn, Maidenhead: Open University Press.

Hellen, N. (2014) Rise of new Underclass Costs £30bn, *The Sunday Times*, 17 August, available at: www.thesundaytimes.co.uk/sto/news/uk_news/Society/article1447828.ece, accessed 18 August 2014.

Hill, K., Sutton, L. and Hirsch, D. (2011) *Living on a Low Income in Later Life: an overview*, London: Age UK.

Hirsch, D. (2006) *Paying for Long-Term Care: moving forward*, York: Joseph Rowntree Foundation.

HM Government (2013) *Working Together to Safeguard Children: a guide to inter-agency working to safeguard and promote the welfare of children*, London: Department for Education.

Holland, S., Tannock, S. and Collicott, H. (2011) Everybody's Business? A research review of the informal safeguarding of other people's children in the UK, *Children & Society*, 25, 406–16.

Holman, B. (1993) *A New Deal for Social Welfare*, Oxford: Lion Publishing.

Holman, R. (1978) *Poverty: explanations of social deprivation*, Oxford: Martin Robertson.

Hooper, C. (2011) Child Maltreatment, Ch. 10 in Bradshaw, J. (ed.) *The Well-being of Children in the UK*, Bristol: Policy Press.

Hooper, C., Gorin, S., Cabral, C. and Dyson, C. (2007) *Living with Hardship 24/7: the diverse experiences of families in poverty in England*, London: The Frank Buttle Trust.

Hough, D. (2013) *Unemployment by Ethnic Background*, Standard Note SN/EP/06385, London: House of Commons Library.

House of Commons Health Committee (2003) *The Victoria Climbié Inquiry Report* (HC570, Sixth Report of Session 2002–3), London: The Stationery Office.

Humphries, B. (2004) An Unacceptable Role for Social Work: implementing immigration policy, *British Journal of Social Work*, 34.1, 93–107.

Hunt, S.J. (2005) *The Life Course: a sociological introduction*, Basingstoke: Palgrave Macmillan.

Hutchinson, D. and Woods, R. (2010) *Children Talking to ChildLine about Loneliness*, Childline Casenotes, London: NSPCC.

Hyde, B. (2013) Mutual Aid Group Work: social work leading the way to recovery-focused mental health practice, *Social Work with Groups*, 36, 43–58.

International Federation of Social Work (IFSW) (2012) *IFSW Policy Statement: health*, Berne: IFSW, available at: http://ifsw.org/policies/health.

Jack, G. (2000) Ecological Influences on Parenting and Child Development, *British Journal of Social Work*, 30, 703–20.

Jack, G. (2004) Child Protection at the Community Level, *Child Abuse Review*, 13, 368–83.

Jack, G. and Gill, O. (2003) *The Missing Side of the Triangle: assessing the importance of family and environmental factors in the lives of children*, Ilford: Barnardo's.

Jack, G. and Gill, O. (2010a) The Impact of Economic Factors on Parents or Caregivers and Children, Ch. 21 in Horwath, J. (ed.) *The Child's World*, 2nd edn, London: Jessica Kingsley.

Jack, G. and Gill, O. (2010b) The Role of Communities in Safeguarding Children and Young People, *Child Abuse Review*, 19, 82–96.

Jack, G. and Gill, O. (2010c) The Impact of Family and Community Support on Parents or Caregivers and Children, Ch. 22 in Horwath, J. (ed.) *The Child's World*, 2nd edn, London: Jessica Kingsley.

Jenkins, S. (2011) *Changing Fortunes: income mobility and poverty dynamics in Britain*, Oxford: Oxford University Press.

Johnson, J. (2002) Taking Care of Later Life: a matter of justice? *British Journal of Social Work*, 32, 739–50.

Jolly, D. (2012) *A Tale of two Models: disabled people vs Unum, Atos, government and disability charities*, Disabled People Against Cuts (DPAC), http://dpac.uk.net/2012/04/a-tale-of-two-models-disabled-people-vs-unum-atos-government-and-disability-charities-debbie-jolly.

Jones, C. (2002) Poverty & Social Exclusion, Ch. 1.1 in Davies, M. (ed.) *The Blackwell Companion to Social Work*, 2nd edn, Oxford: Blackwell.

Jones, C. and Novak, T. (1999) *Poverty, Welfare and the Disciplinary State*, London: Routledge.

Jones, C., Ferguson, I., Lavalette, M. and Penketh, L. (2007) Social Work and Social Justice: a manifesto for a new engaged practice, Ch. 11 in Lavalette, M. and Ferguson, I. (eds) *International Social Work and the Radical Tradition*, Birmingham: Venture Press.

Jordan, B. (2012) Foreword, in Rogowski, S. (2013) *Critical Social Work with Children and Families: theory, context and practice*, Bristol: Policy Press.

Jordan, B. and Drakeford, M. (2012) *Social Work and Social Policy under Austerity*, Basingstoke: Palgrave Macmillan.

Joseph Rowntree Foundation (2004) *Older People Shaping Policy and Practice*, York: Joseph Rowntree Foundation.

Joyce, R. and Sibieta, L. (2013) *Labour's Record on Poverty and Inequality*, London: Institute for Fiscal Studies, available at: www.ifs.org.uk/publications/6738.

Karban, K. (2011) *Social Work and Mental Health*, Cambridge: Polity Press.

Kaye, A., Jordan, H. and Baker, M. (2012) *The Tipping Point: the human and economic costs of cutting disabled people's support*, Hardest Hit coalition, available at: http://thehardesthit.wordpress.com/our-message/the-tipping-point.

Keating, F. (2007) *African and Caribbean Men and Mental Health*, Better Health Briefing 5, London: Race Equality Foundation.

Keating, F., Robertson, D., McCulloch, A. and Francis, E. (2002) *Breaking the Circles of Fear*, London: Sainsbury Centre for Mental Health.

Kenway, P. and Palmer, G. (2007) *Poverty Among Ethnic Groups: how and why does it differ?* York: Joseph Rowntree Foundation.

Kerr, B., Gordon, J., MacDonald, C. and Stalker, K. (2005) *Effective Social Work with Older People*, Edinburgh: Scottish Executive.

Kneale, D. (2012) *Is Social Exclusion Still Important for Older People?* London: International Longevity Centre.

Kreiger, N. (1999) Embodying Inequality: a review of concepts, measures, and methods for studying health consequences of discrimination, *International Journal of Health Services*, 29.2, 295–352.

Lavalette, M. and Ferguson, I. (eds) (2007) *International Social Work and the Radical Tradition*, Birmingham: Venture Press.

Law, I. (2012) Poverty and Income Maintenance, Ch. 10 in Craig, G., Atkin, K., Chattoo, S. and Flynn, R. (eds) *Understanding 'Race' and Ethnicity: theory, history, policy, practice*, Bristol: Policy Press.

Lawrence, F. (2008) Britain on a Plate, *The Guardian*, 1 October, available at: www.guardian.co.uk/lifeandstyle/2008/oct/01/foodanddrink.oliver, accessed 6 December 2010.

Leader, D. (2011) *What is Madness?* London: Hamish Hamilton.

Ledwith, M. (1997) Community Development: a critical approach, Bristol: BASW/Policy Press.

Lee, E., Clements, S., Ingham, R. and Stone, N. (2004) *A Matter of Choice? Explaining national variation in teenage abortion and motherhood*, York: Joseph Rowntree Foundation.

Levitas, R. (2005) *The Inclusive Society? Social exclusion and New Labour*, 2nd edn, Basingstoke: Palgrave Macmillan.

Levitas, R. (2012a) The Just's Umbrella: austerity and the Big Society in coalition policy and beyond, *Critical Social Policy*, 32.3, 320–42.

Levitas, R. (2012b) There May Be 'Trouble' Ahead: what we know about those 120,000 'troubled' families, *Poverty and Social Exclusion*, available at: www.poverty.ac.uk/report-housing-living-standards-income-distribution-low-income-households-employment-families/flaws.

Levitas, R., Pantazis, C., Fahmy, E., Gordon, D., Lloyd, E. and Patsios, D. (2007) *The Multi-dimensional Analysis of Social Exclusion*, Bristol: University of Bristol.

Link, B. and Phelan, J. (2001) Conceptualizing Stigma, *Annual Review of Sociology*, 27, 363–85.

Lister, R. (2004) *Poverty*, Cambridge: Polity Press.

Lloyd, L. (2006) A Caring Profession? The ethics of care and social work with older people, *British Journal of Social Work*, 36, 1171–85.

Lonne, B., Parton, N., Thomson, J. and Harries M. (2009) *Reforming Child Protection*, Abingdon: Routledge.

Low, J. (2011) *The Riots: what are the lessons from the JRF's work in communities?* (summary), York: Joseph Rowntree Foundation.

Lupton, R. and Kneale, D. (2010) *Are there Neighbourhood Effects on Teenage Parenthood in the UK, and Does it Matter for Policy? A review of theory and evidence*, London: Centre for Analysis of Social Exclusion.

Lymbery, M. (2001) Social Work at the Crossroads, *British Journal of Social Work*, 31.3, 369–84.

Lymbery, M. (2004) Responding to the Crisis: the changing nature of welfare organisation, Ch. 2 in Lymbery, M. and Butler, S. (eds) *Social Work Ideals and Practice Realities*, Basingstoke: Palgrave Macmillan.

Lymbery, M. and Butler, S. (eds) (2004) *Social Work Ideals and Practice Realities*, Basingstoke: Palgrave Macmillan.

Lynch, R. (2014) *Social Work with Older People: a positive person-centred approach*, London: Sage.

Lyons, J. (2014) Killed by Benefits Cuts: starving soldier died 'as result of Iain Duncan Smith's welfare reform', *The Mirror*, 27 July, available at: http://www.mirror.co.uk/news/uk-news/killed-benefits-cuts-starving-soldier-3923771#ixzz39nP99xBu, accessed 8 August 2014.

MacInnes, T., Aldridge, H., Bushe, S., Kenway, P. and Tinson, A. (2013) *Monitoring Poverty and Social Exclusion 2013*, York: Joseph Rowntree Foundation.

Manthorpe, J., Moriarty, J., Rapaport, J., Clough, R., Cornes, M., Bright, L., Iliffe, S. and OPRSI (Older People Researching Social Issues) (2008) 'There Are Wonderful Social Workers but it's a Lottery': older people's views about social workers, *British Journal of Social Work*, 38, 1132–50.

Marmot, M. (2004) *Status Syndrome: how your social standing directly affects your health and life expectancy*, London: Bloomsbury.

Marmot Review Team (2010) *Fair Society, Healthy Lives: the Marmot Review*, strategic review of health inequalities in England post 2010, London: The Marmot Review.

McDermott, D. (2014) The Problem with Recovery, in Weinstein, J. (ed.) *Mental Health*, Bristol: Policy Press.

McLaughlin, K. (2005) From Ridicule to Institutionalization: anti-oppression, the state and social work, *Critical Social Policy*, 25.3, 283–305.

McManus, S., Meltzer, H., Brugha, T., Bebbington, P. and Jenkins, R. (2009) *Adult Psychiatric Morbidity in England, 2007: results of a household survey*, London: National Centre for Social Research.

McNeil, C. and Hunter, J. (2014) *The Generation Strain: collective solutions to care in an ageing society*, London: Institute for Public Policy Research.

Meltzer, H., Singleton, S., Lee, A., Bebbington, P., Brugha, T. and Jenkins R. (2002) *The Social and Economic Circumstances of Adults with Mental Disorders*, London: TSO.

Millar, J. (2009) The United Kingdom: the feminization of poverty? Ch. 5 in Schaffner Goldberg, G. (2009) *Poor Women in Rich Countries: the feminization of poverty over the life course*, Oxford: Oxford University Press.

Monroe, J. (2012) Hunger Hurts, *A Girl Called Jack*, (blog), available at: http://agirlcalledjack.com/2012/07/30/hunger-hurts/.

Mooney, G. (1998) Remoralizing the Poor? Gender, class & philanthropy in Victorian Britain, Ch. 2 in Lewis, G. (ed.) *Forming Nation, Framing Welfare*, London: Routledge/Open University.

Moosa, Z. with Woodroffe, J. (2009) *Poverty Pathways: ethnic minority women's livelihoods*, London: Fawcett Society/Oxfam.

Morgan, T. (2011) *'I buy, therefore I am': the economic meaning of the riots*, Tullett Prebon strategy notes, Issue 24, London: Tullett Prebon.

Morris, D. and Gilchrist, A. (2011) *Communities Connected: inclusion, participation and common purpose*, London: Royal Society for the encouragement of Arts, Manufactures and Commerce.

Morris, J. (2011) *Rethinking Disability Policy*, York: Joseph Rowntree Foundation.

Munn-Giddings, C. and McVicar, A. (2006) Self-help Groups as Mutual Support: what do carers value? *Health and Social Care in the Community*, 15.1, 26–34.

Munro, E. (2011) *The Munro Review of Child Protection: final report. A child-centred system*, Cm. 8062, London: Department for Education.

Munro, E. (2012) *The Munro Review of Child Protection: progress report: moving towards a child centred system*, London: Department for Education.

Murali, V. and Oyebode, F. (2004) Poverty, social inequality and mental health, *Advances in Psychiatric Treatment*, 10, 216–24.

Murray, C. (1989) The Emerging British Underclass, in Murray, C. (1996) *Charles Murray and the Underclass: the developing debate*, London: IEA Health and Welfare Unit in association with *The Sunday Times*.

Murray, C. (1990) Rejoinder, in Murray, C. (1996) *Charles Murray and the Underclass: the developing debate*, London: IEA Health and Welfare Unit in association with *The Sunday Times*.

National Equality Panel (2010) *An Anatomy of Economic Inequality in the UK: report of the National Equality Panel*, CASE Report 60, London: Government Equalities Office and Centre for Analysis of Social Exclusion, London School of Economics.

National Evaluation of Sure Start Team (2012) *The impact of Sure Start Local Programmes on Seven Year Olds and their Families*, London: Department for Education.

Nazroo, J., Bejekal, M., Blane, D. and Grewal, I. (2004) Ethnic Inequalities, Ch. 3 in Walker, A. and Hennessy, C.H. (eds) *Growing Older: quality of life in old age*, Maidenhead: Open University Press.

NICE (National Institute for Health and Care Excellence) (2013) *Antisocial Behaviour and Conduct Disorders in Children and Young People: recognition, intervention and management*, NICE Clinical Guideline 158, Manchester: NICE.

Novak, T. (1988) *Poverty and the State*, Milton Keynes: Open University Press.

NSUN (2012), *No Health Without Mental Health: a guide for service users*, London: NSUN.

Nwabuzo, O. (2012) *The Riot Roundtables: race and the riots of August 2011*, London: Runnymede Trust.

Nyabingi (2011) *Profile of Nyabingi*, Luton: Nyabingi.

O'Hagan, M. (2002) Living Well, *Openmind*, 118, 16–17.

O'Hagan, M. (2012) Recovery: is consensus possible? *World Psychiatry*, 11.3, 167–8.

Ofcom (2013) *Communications Market Report 2013*, London: Ofcom.

Oliver, M. (2009) *Understanding Disability: from theory to practice*, 2nd edn, Basingstoke: Palgrave Macmillan.

Oliver, M. and Barnes, C. (2012) *The New Politics of Disablement*, Basingstoke: Palgrave Macmillan.

Oliver, M., Sapey, B. and Thomas, P. (2012) *Social Work with Disabled People*, Basingstoke: Palgrave Macmillan.

ONS (2012a) *Mortality in England and Wales: average life span*, London: ONS.

ONS (2012b) *Population Ageing in the United Kingdom, its Constituent Countries and the European Union*, London: ONS.

ONS (2012c) *Pension Trends*, London: ONS.

ONS (2013a) *Poverty and Social Exclusion in the UK and EU, 2005–2011*, London: ONS.

ONS (2013b) *Disability in England and Wales, 2011 and Comparison with 2001*, London: ONS.

ONS (2013c) *Full Story: the gender gap in unpaid care provision: is there an impact on health and economic position?* London: ONS.

Orwell, G. (1987) *Nineteen Eighty-four*, London: Secker & Warburg, first published 1949.

Osborne, G. and Duncan Smith, I. (2012) George Osborne and Iain Duncan Smith set out how they will end the 'something for nothing' culture, *Daily Mail*, 8 October, available at: www.dailymail.co.uk/news/article-2214384/George-Osborne-Iain-Duncan-Smith-set-end-culture.html.

Overton, S. and Medina, S. (2008) The Stigma of Mental Illness, *Journal of Counseling & Development*, 86, 143–51.

Owen, C. and Statham, J. (2009) *Disproportionality in Child Welfare: the prevalence of black and minority ethnic children within the 'looked after' and 'children in need' populations and on Child Protection Registers in England*, London: Department for Children, Schools and Families.

Palmer, G. (2006) Disabled People, Poverty and the Labour Market, in Preston, G. (ed.) *A Route out of Poverty? Disabled people, work and welfare reform*, London: Child Poverty Action Group.

Palmer, G. (2011) Working-age Out-of-work Benefit Recipients, *The Poverty Site*, available at: www.poverty.org.uk/13/index.shtml.

Parekh, A., MacInnes, T. and Kenway, P. (2010) *Monitoring Poverty and Social Exclusion 2010*, York: Joseph Rowntree Foundation/New Policy Institute.

Parrott, L. (2014) *Social Work and Poverty: a critical approach*, Bristol: Policy Press.

Parsonage, M., Khan, L. and Saunders, A. (2014) *Building a Better Future: the lifetime costs of childhood behavioural problems and the benefits of early intervention*, London: Centre for Mental Health.

Parton, N. (2011) Child Protection and Safeguarding in England: changing and competing conceptions of risk and their implications for social work, *British Journal of Social Work*, 41.5, 854–75.

Parton, N. (2012) The Munro Review of Child Protection: an appraisal, *Children and Society*, 26, 150–62.

Patrick, R. (2012) Work as the Primary 'Duty' of the Responsible Citizen: a critique of this work-centric approach, *People, Place & Policy Online*, 6.1, 5–15.

Paxman, J. (2011) 'I am part of the most selfish generation in history and we should be ashamed of our legacy', *Daily Mail*, 31 October, available at: www.dailymail.co.uk/news/article-2055497/JEREMY-PAXMAN-Baby-Boomers-selfish-generation-history.html, accessed 6 March 2013.

Pembroke, L. (1996) It Helped that Someone Believed Me, in Read, J. and Reynolds, J. (eds) *Speaking Our Minds*, Basingstoke: Macmillan.

Perry, N. (ed.) (2005) *Getting the Right Trainers: enabling service users to train social work students and practitioners about the realities of family poverty in the UK*, London: ATD Fourth World.

Pickles, C. (2010) Repairing the Broken Society: the way forward, *Journal of Poverty and Social Justice*, 18.2, 161–6.

Pierson, J. (2008) *Going Local: working in communities and neighbourhoods*, London: Routledge.

Pierson, J. (2010) *Tackling Social Exclusion*, 2nd edn, London: Routledge.

Platt, L. (2009) *Ethnicity and Child Poverty*, Research Report No 576, London: Department for Work and Pensions.

Preston, G. (2005) *Hard-working Families: caring for two or more disabled children*, London: Disability Alliance.

Preston, G. (ed.) (2006) *A Route Out of Poverty? Disabled people, work and welfare reform*, London: Child Poverty Action Group.

Price, D. (2006) The Poverty of Older People in the UK, *Journal of Social Work Practice*, 20.3, 251–66.

Priestley, M. (2000) Adults Only: disability, social policy and the life course, *Journal of Social Policy*, 29.3, 421–39.

PSE (Poverty and Social Exclusion) (2013) What do we Think we Need? *PSE Research*, available at: www.poverty.ac.uk/pse-research/3-what-do-we-think-we-need, accessed 13 May 2013.

Public Accounts Committee (2013) *Department for Work and Pensions: management of contract medical services*, 23rd Report of Session 2012–13, HC 744, London: The Stationery Office.

Radford, L., Corral, S., Bradley, C., Fisher, H., Bassett, C., Howat, N. and Collishaw, S. (2011) *Child Abuse and Neglect in the UK Today*, London: NSPCC.

Rajan-Rankin, S. and Beresford, P. (2011) *Critical Observations on the Munro Review of Child Protection*, Social Work Action Network, available at: www.socialworkfuture.org/articles-and-analysis/analysis/sw-taskforce/150-munro-review-critique.

Ray, M. and Phillips, J. (2012) *Social Work with Older People*, 5th edn, Basingstoke: Palgrave Macmillan.

Read, J. and Baker, S. (1996) *Not Just Sticks & Stones: a survey of the stigma, taboos and discrimination experienced by people with mental health problems*, London: Mind.

Reed, H. (2012) *In the Eye of the Storm: Britain's forgotten children and families*, London: Action for Children, The Children's Society and NSPCC.

Refugee Council (2006) *The Destitution Trap: research into destitution among refused asylum seekers in the UK*, London: Refugee Council.

Richardson, B. (ed.) (2007) *Tell It Like It Is: how our schools fail Black children*, 2nd edn, London: Bookmarks.

Ridge, T. and Millar, J. (2011) Following Families: working lone mother families and their children, *Social Policy & Administration*, 45.1, 85–97.

Riots, Communities and Victims Panel (RCVP) (2012) *After the Riots: the final report of the Riots Communities and Victims Panel*, London: RCVP.

Rodrigues, L. (2103) *Food for Thought: a survey of teachers' views on school meals*, London: The Children's Society.

Rogers, A. and Pilgrim, D. (2010) *A Sociology of Mental Health and Illness*, 4th edn, Maidenhead: Open University Press.

Rogowski, S. (2013) *Critical Social Work with Children and Families: theory, context and practice*, Bristol: Policy Press.

Rose, S.M. and Hatzenbuehler, S. (2009) Embodying Social Class: the link between poverty, income inequality and health, *International Social Work*, 52.4, 459–71.

Rose, W. (2010) The Assessment Framework, Ch. 2 in Horwath, J. (ed.) *The Child's World*, 2nd edn, London: Jessica Kingsley.

Rowlingson, K. (2011) *Does Income Inequality Cause Health and Social Problems?* York: Joseph Rowntree Foundation.

Rowntree, B.S. (2000) *Poverty: a study of town life*, Bristol: Policy Press, first published 1901.

Royal College of Psychiatrists (Social Inclusion Scoping Group) (2009) *Mental Health and Social Inclusion: making psychiatry and mental health services fit for the 21st century*, London: Royal College of Psychiatrists.

Salvation Army (2004) *The Responsibility Gap: individualism, community and responsibility in Britain today*, London: Salvation Army/Henley Centre.

Salway, S., Platt, L., Chowbey, P., Harriss, K. and Bayliss, E. (2007) *Long-term Ill Health, Poverty and Ethnicity*, Bristol: Policy Press/Joseph Rowntree Foundation.

Sanis, N. (2010) *Championing the Extended Schools Social Worker Role: prevention and practice*, Leeds: Children's Workforce Development Council.

Scharf, T., Phillipson, C. and Smith, A.E. (2004) Poverty and Social Exclusion: growing older in deprived urban neighbourhoods, Ch. 5 in Walker, A. and Hennessy, C.H. (eds) *Growing Older: quality of life in old age*, Maidenhead: Open University Press.

SCIE (2012) *Introduction to Adult Mental Health Services*, London: SCIE.

SCIE (2013) *Social Work Practice Pilots and Pioneers in Social Work for Adults*, London: SCIE.

Scott, K., Booth, R. and Harding, L. (2010) Red Road Deaths: a tragedy of asylum, mental health and Russian intrigue, *The Guardian*, 12 March, available at: www.guardian.co.uk/uk/2010/mar/12/red-road-deaths-russian-asylum-seekers, accessed 18 June 2010.

Seabrook, J. (2003) *The No-Nonsense Guide to World Poverty*, Oxford and London: New Internationalist Publications/Verso.

Secretary of State for Work and Pensions (2010) *21st Century Welfare*, Cm 7913, London: The Stationery Office.

Secretary of State for Work and Pensions (2012) *Social Justice: transforming lives*, Cm 8314, London: The Stationery Office.

Seebohm Report (1968) *Report of the Committee on Local Authority and Allied Personal Social Services*, Cmnd 3703, London: HMSO.

Seebohm, P., Gilchrist, A. and Morris, D. (2012) Bold but Balanced: how community development contributes to mental health and inclusion, *Community Development Journal*, 47.4, 473–90.

Sen, A. (1987) The Standard of Living: lecture II, lives and capabilities, in Hawthorn. G. (ed.) *The Standard of Living*, Cambridge: Cambridge University Press.

SETF (2007a) *Reaching Out: progress on social exclusion*, London: Cabinet Office.

SETF (2007b) *Reaching Out: think family: analysis and themes from the Families at Risk Review*, London: Cabinet Office.

SEU (1999) *Teenage Pregnancy*, London: HMSO.

SEU (2001) *Preventing Social Exclusion*, London: SEU.

SEU (2004) *Mental Health and Social Exclusion*, London: Office of the Deputy Prime Minister.

SEU (2006) *A Sure Start to Later Life: ending inequalities for older people*, London: Office of the Deputy Prime Minister.

Sewell, H. and Waterhouse, S. (2012) *Making Progress on Race Equality in Mental Health*, London: NHS Confederation, Mental Health Network.

Sheldon, B. and Macdonald, G. (2009) *A Textbook of Social Work*, London: Routledge.

Shepherd, G., Boardman, J. and Slade, M. (2008) *Making Recovery a Reality*, London: Sainsbury Centre for Mental Health.

Sheppard, M. (2006) *Social Work and Social Exclusion: the idea of practice*, Aldershot: Ashgate.

Shildrick, T., MacDonald Webster, C. and Garthwaite, K. (2012) *Poverty and Insecurity: life in low-pay, no-pay Britain*, Bristol: Policy Press.

Smedley, T. (2013) Malnutrition Among the Elderly: task force calls for national strategy, *Guardian Professional*, 31 May.

Smith, M. (2013) Anti-stigma Campaigns: time to change, editorial, *British Journal of Psychiatry*, 202: s49–50.

Smith, N. and Middleton, S. (2007) *A Review of Poverty Dynamics Research in the UK*, York: Joseph Rowntree Foundation.

Smith, N., Middleton, S., Ashton-Brooks, K., Cox, L. and Dobson, B. with Reith, L. (2004) *Disabled People's Costs of Living: 'more than you would think'*, York: Joseph Rowntree Foundation.

Smith, R. (2012) Life Beyond the Council: meet the social work pioneers, *Community Care*, 21 August, available at: www.communitycare.co.uk/2012/08/21/life-beyond-the-council-meet-the-social-work-pioneers, accessed 18 August 2014.

Sparrow, A. (2010) Parental 'Warmth' More Important than Wealth, says David Cameron, *The Guardian*, available at: www.guardian.co.uk/politics/2010/jan/11/david-cameron-nature-v-nurture, accessed, 11 April 2013.

Spartacus (2012) *The People's Review of the Work Capability Assessment*, We are Spartacus, available at: http://wearespartacus.org.uk/wca-report.

Spencer, N. and Baldwin, N. (2005) Economic, Cultural and Social Contexts of Neglect, Ch. 2 in Taylor, J. and Daniel, B. (eds) *Child Neglect: practice issues for health and social care*, London: Jessica Kingsley.

Spicker, P. (2007) *The Idea of Poverty*, Bristol: Policy Press.

Stein, M. (2006) Research Review: young people leaving care, *Child and Family Social Work*, 11.3, 273–9.

Steinberg, D.M. (2014) *A Mutual-Aid Model for Social Work with Groups*, 3rd edn, London: Routledge.

Stepney, P. and Popple, K. (2008) *Social Work and the Community: a critical context for practice*, Basingstoke: Palgrave Macmillan.

Stewart, K. (2012) Child Poverty: what have we really achieved? Ch. 1 in Judge, L. (ed.) *Ending Child Poverty by 2020: progress made and lessons learned*, London: Child Poverty Action Group.

Strelitz, J. and Lister, R. (eds) (2008) *Why Money Matters: family income, poverty and children's lives*, London: Save the Children.

Strier, R. and Binyamin, S. (2010) Developing Anti-Oppressive Services for the Poor: a theoretical and organisational rationale, *British Journal of Social Work*, 40, 1908–26.

SWAN (2010) *Privatization of Children's services: independent 'social work practices'*, Midlands Social Work Action Network Briefing, Paisley: SWAN.

Tanner, D. and Harris, J. (2007) *Working with Older People*, London: Routledge/Community Care.

Taylor, D. (2009) *Underground Lives*, Leeds: PAFRAS.

Teater, T. and Baldwin, M. (2012) *Social Work in the Community: making a difference*, Bristol: Policy Press/BASW.

Tew, J. (2011) *Social Approaches to Mental Distress*, Basingstoke: Palgrave Macmillan.

Tew, J., Ramon, S., Slade, M., Bird, V., Melton, J. and Le Boutillier, C. (2011) Social Factors and Recovery from Mental Health Difficulties: a review of the evidence, *British Journal of Social Work*, 42.3, 443–60.

The College of Social Work (2012) *Domains Within the PCF*, London: The College of Social Work.

The College of Social Work (2013) *Code of Ethics for Membership of The College of Social Work*, London: The College of Social Work.

The College of Social Work (2014) *Social Work with Adults: what does the future hold?* London: The College of Social Work.

Thompson, N. (2012) *Anti-discriminatory Practice: equality, diversity and social justice*, 5th edn, Basingstoke: Palgrave Macmillan.

Time to Change (2012) *Children and Young People's Programme Development: summary of research and insights*, London: Time to Change.

Tomlinson, M. and Walker, R. (2009) *Coping with Complexity: child and adult poverty*, London: CPAG.

Tomlinson, M. and Walker, R. (2010) *Recurrent Poverty: the impact of family and labour market changes*, York: Joseph Rowntree Foundation.

Townsend, P. (1979) *Poverty in the United Kingdom: a survey of household resources and standards of living*, Harmondsworth: Penguin.

Townsend, P. and Davidson, N. (eds) (1982) *Inequalities in Health: The Black Report*, Harmondsworth: Penguin, available at: www.sochealth.co.uk/history/black.htm.

UCL Institute of Health Equity (2012) *The Impact of the Economic Downturn and Policy Changes on Health Inequalities in London*, London: UCL Institute of Health Equity.

United Nations (2005) *The Inequality Predicament: report on the world social situation*, New York: United Nations.

Utting, D. (ed.) (2009) *Contemporary Social Evils*, Bristol: Policy Press/Joseph Rowntree Foundation.

Walker, A. (1990) Blaming the Victims, in Murray, C. (1996) *Charles Murray and the Underclass: the developing debate*, London: IEA Health and Welfare Unit in association with *The Sunday Times*.

Wallcraft, J., Read, J. and Sweeney, A. (2003) *On Our Own Terms: users and survivors of mental health services working together for support and change*, London: Sainsbury Centre for Mental Health.

Wanless, D. (2006) *Securing Good Care for Older People: taking a long-term view*, London: King's Fund.

War on Want (2006) *The Global Workplace: challenging the race to the bottom – a manual for trade union activists*, London: War on Want.

Welbourne, P. (2012) *Social Work with Children and Families*, London: Routledge.

White, V. (2009) Quiet Challenges? Professional practice in modernised social work, Ch. 7 in Harris, J. and White, V. (eds) *Modernising Social Work: critical considerations*, Bristol: Policy Press.

WHO (2007) *Breaking the Vicious Cycle Between Mental Ill-health and Poverty* (information sheet), Geneva: WHO.

Wilkinson, R. (1996) *Unhealthy Societies: the afflictions of inequality*, London: Routledge.

Wilkinson, R. and Pickett, K. (2009) *The Spirit Level: why more equal societies almost always do better*, London: Allen Lane.

Wilks, T. (2012) *Advocacy and Social Work Practice*, Maidenhead: Open University Pres.

Williams, Z. (2014) Whose Fault is Poverty? The election blame game is on, *The Guardian*, available at: www.theguardian.com/society/2014/aug/03/victims-britains-harsh-welfare-sanctions, accessed 18 August 2014.

Wintour, P. (2011) Employment Benefit Test Finds Two-thirds of Claimants Fit for Work, *The Guardian*, available at: www.guardian.co.uk/uk/2011/jul/26/employment-allowance-test-discriminates-disabled.

Women's Aid (2008) Providing Support for 'Children in Need': Section 17 of the Children Act 1989, available at: www.womensaid.org.uk/domestic-violence-articles.asp?section=00010001002200020001 &itemid=1450, accessed 23 April 2013.

Women's Budget Group (2005) *Women's and Children's Poverty: making the links*, London: Women's Budget Group.

Wood, C., Salter, J., Morrell, G., Barnes, M., Paget, A. and O'Leary, D. (2012) *Poverty in Perspective*, London: Demos.

Index

accessing services 84–5
accumulation of risk model, life course perspective 64
adolescents, mental distress 116, 121
ageing society 100–4
ageism 97–8, 100–4
agency, cultural theories of poverty 25–9
anti-poverty practice 89–95
assessments 167, 168–9
　Common Assessment Framework (CAF) 93–4
　needs assessment 156–7
　Work Capability Assessment 46–8
asylum seekers 1, 90, 162, 166
austerity policies 4–6

black and minority ethnic (BME) groups
　child abuse 77–8
　Disability Living Allowance (DLA) 43
　ethnic poverty penalty 41–3
　gender issues 42
　intersectionality 41, 42
　mental distress 128–31, 135–6
　old age 103–4
　population growth 103–4
　poverty 24–5
　rioting 55–6
　risk factors of poverty 42
　settlement pattern 40
　social exclusion 40–3
The Black Report (1982) 57–8
Blair, Tony 33, 52
blaming people for their own poverty 13, 34–5
BME *see* black and minority ethnic groups
'Broken Britain' 51–7

CAF *see* Common Assessment Framework
Cameron, David
　disability 47
　rioting 56, 71
　teenage pregnancy/parenthood 69–70
　'Troubled Families' 36
capabilities framework, disability 48–9
capitalism 23
care management, old age 108–13
carers 104–5
　social workers 105
Centre for Social Justice 112
Charity Organization Society (COS) 11–13

child abuse 76–81
　see also domestic violence
　black and minority ethnic (BME) groups 77–8
　defining 81
　Every Child Matters 78, 82, 83, 85, 90
　gender issues 77
　neglect 78–80
　poverty 76–81
　preventing 81–5, 89, 90, 95
　protecting 81–2, 85, 87, 89, 93–5
　safeguarding 81, 84–5, 90, 93, 95
　Victoria Climbié case 54, 77–8
children's health
　health inequalities 61–5
　life course 63–5
coalition government 4–5, 22, 23–4, 29
　State of the Nation 38
　teenage pregnancy/parenthood 66, 69–71
　'Troubled Families' 36–7, 90
　Work Capability Assessment 46–7
Common Assessment Framework (CAF) 93–4
communities transformation 53
Community Care Act 1990: 109
community needs profiling 156–7
community-orientated vs. traditional approaches to social work 153
community social work (CSW) 149–54, 169
　social inclusion 151
conduct disorders 121, 123–4
COS *see* Charity Organization Society
countries comparison, UNICEF 'Report Card' 71–2
credit unions 26–7
critical period model
　life course perspective 64
CSW *see* community social work
cultural theories of poverty 23–5
　agency 25–9

de-industrialization 52–3
demographic time bomb/transition 100–1
'deserving' and 'undeserving' cases 12–14, 19–20, 140–1
disability 43–9
　barriers 45–6
　capabilities framework 48–9
　discourses of exclusion 47
　Employment and Support Allowance (ESA) 46
　Households Below Average Income (HBAI) 43

disability (contd.)
  vs. illness 45
  vs. impairment 44–5
  individual model 48–9
  Job Seekers' Allowance (JSA) 46
  risk factors 102
  self-respect 44
  social exclusion 43–9
  social inequalities 44
  social model 48–9
  Work Capability Assessment 46–8
Disability Living Allowance (DLA) 43, 46
discretion vs. managerial control, social work
      practice 146–9
discrimination
  mental distress 125–8
  personal, cultural and structural (PCS) model 127
DLA see Disability Living Allowance
domestic violence 61–3, 77, 90–2
  see also child abuse
  social care resources 142
Doublethink 161, 162, 164, 165
drapetomania 120

education, social work 8–9
Employment and Support Allowance (ESA) 46
empowering children
  teamwork approach 94
empowering options 142
ESA see Employment and Support Allowance
ethical dimension
  poverty 7
ethics and values 143–5
ethnic minorities see black and minority ethnic
      (BME) groups
ethnic poverty penalty 41–3
ethnicity, mental distress 128–31
Every Child Matters 78, 82, 83, 85, 90

Fair Access to Care Services (FACS) bandings
      110, 171–2
  eligibility criteria 171–2
family poverty 90–2, 164
feminization of poverty 25, 66
Field MP, Frank 35, 70–1
food banks 5, 141, 162, 163

gender issues
  black and minority ethnic (BME) groups 42
  child abuse 77
globalization 52–5
  social work practice 55
group work
  mental distress 134–7
growth of poverty 23–5

HBAI see Households Below Average Income
health determinant, social status 71–2
health inequalities 6
  The Black Report (1982) 57–8
  children's health 61–5
  domestic violence 61–3
  social work 57–65
homosexuality 120
Households Below Average Income (HBAI) 18–19
  disability 43

illness, vs. disability 45
impairment, vs. disability 44–5
individual model, disability 48–9
inequality, mental distress 116–17, 128–31
institutional racism 131–2
  defining 131

Job Seekers' Allowance (JSA) 46
Joseph Rowntree Foundation (JRF) 53–4
JSA see Job Seekers' Allowance

Labour government 4, 7, 19, 32–3
  Social Exclusion Unit (SEU) 35
  Teenage Pregnancy Strategy 39, 66–7
life course 63–5
Living with Hardship study 78–9
loneliness, old age 106

managerial control vs. discretion, social work
      practice 146–9
measuring poverty 14–20, 29
mental distress 115–37
  adolescents 116
  black and minority ethnic (BME) groups 128–31,
      135–6
  causes 116–17
  conduct disorders 121, 123–4
  defining 119
  discrimination 125–8
  drapetomania 120
  ethnicity 128–31
  functional disorders 118
  group work 134–7
  homosexuality 120
  inequality 116–17, 128–31
  institutional racism 131–2
  life course perspectives 122–3
  medical model 119–20
  mutual aid 134–7
  poverty 116–17
  recovery 132–4
  social exclusion 117–18
  social model of madness 122–5
  social realism 120

stigma 125–8
  'toxic trio' 124–5
MUD (moral underclass discourse) 37
The Munro Review of Child Protection 89
mutual aid 169
  defining 134–5
  mental distress 134–7
mutuality, ethics and values 144–5

needs assessment 156–7
neglect 62
  child abuse 78–80
  defining 78
  vs. poverty 76–80, 163
neighbourhood effects
  defining 38
  old age 105–8
  social exclusion 38–9

old age
  ageism 97–8, 100–4
  black and minority ethnic (BME) groups 103–4
  care management 108–13
  carers 104–5
  Community Care Act 1990: 109
  complexity of interrelated factors 107–8
  digital divide 103
  Fair Access to Care Services (FACS) bandings 110
  loneliness 106
  neighbourhood effects 105–8
  privatization of services 109–10
  social exclusion 98–9
  social isolation 105–6
  A Sure Start to Later Life 110
outline of this book 9–10

parenting 66–74
  see also teenage pregnancy/parenthood
political influence 4–6
poverty
  black and minority ethnic (BME) groups 24–5
  capitalism 23
  causes 21–5, 28–9
  child abuse 76–81
  cultural theories 23–5
  defining 2–3, 8, 14–16
  ethical dimension 7
  family poverty 90–2, 164
  feminization of poverty 25
  growth of poverty 23–5
  impact 1–3, 7
  Living with Hardship study 78–9
  measuring 14–20, 29
  mental distress 116–17

vs. neglect 76–80, 163
  pathological theories 21–3
  psychological impact 7
  relative poverty 14–20
  'root causes' 24
  vs. social exclusion 2–3
  social exclusion 90–2
  social support 80
  structural theories 23–5
poverty blindness 1–2
poverty dynamics 27–9
povertyism 13–14
pregnancy, teenage *see* teenage pregnancy/
    parenthood
privatization of services, old age 109–10
psychological impact of poverty 7

recovery, mental distress 132–4
RED (redistribution discourse) 37
relative poverty 14–20
'Right Trainers' project 8
rioting and social inequalities 55–7
risk factors of poverty
  black and minority ethnic (BME) groups 42
at risk groups, social exclusion 85–8, 90

SCIE *see* Social Care Institute for Excellence
self-esteem, accessing services 84–5
self-respect, disability 44–5
self-stigma 127–8
sensory impairment
  social inclusion 154–6
SETF *see* Social Exclusion Task Force
SEU *see* Social Exclusion Unit
SID (social integrationist discourse) 37
social care approaches 111–13
Social Care Institute for Excellence (SCIE) 152
'social evils' 53–4
social exclusion 35–8
  black and minority ethnic (BME) groups 40–3
  causes 86–8
  challenges 4
  characteristics 2–4
  defining 35, 38
  disability 43–9
  domestic violence 90–2
  mental distress 117–18
  multi-dimensional aspect 32
  neighbourhood effects 38–9
  vs. poverty 2–3
  poverty 90–2
  at risk groups 85–8, 90
  teenage pregnancy/parenthood 68–9
  underclass debate 33–5
Social Exclusion Task Force (SETF) 86–8

Social Exclusion Unit (SEU) 35
  teenage pregnancy/parenthood 66–7
social inclusion
  community social work (CSW) 151
  sensory impairment 154–6
social inequalities
  disability 44
  issues 52
  rioting 55–7
social isolation, old age 105–6
social model, disability 48–9
social model of madness 122–5
social realism 120
social status, health determinant 71–2
social support 80
social work and health inequalities 57–65
social work education 8–9
social work practice
  context 162
  discretion vs. managerial control 146–9
  globalization 55
  traditional vs. community-orientated
      approaches 153
social workers 106–9, 111
  attitude to carers 105
  Centre for Social Justice 112
  challenges 161
  focus 161–2
The Spirit Level 72–3
SSLPs *see* Sure Start Local Programmes
State of the Nation 38

Status Syndrome 72, 73
stigma 13–14, 165
  accessing services 84–5
  mental distress 125–8
  self-stigma 127–8
Sure Start Local Programmes (SSLPs) 82, 83–5
A Sure Start to Later Life 110

teamwork approach, empowering children 94
teenage pregnancy/parenthood 34–5, 39, 66–74
  coalition government 66, 69–71
  social exclusion 68–9
  Social Exclusion Unit (SEU) 66–7
Teenage Pregnancy Strategy, Labour government
      39, 66–7
TOPAZ 152
'toxic trio', mental distress 124–5
traditional vs. community-orientated approaches to
      social work 153
'Troubled Families' 36–7, 90

underclass debate 33–5
UNICEF 'Report Card', countries comparison
      71–2

values and ethics 143–5
Victoria Climbié case, child abuse 54, 77–8
violence, domestic 61–3
visual impairment, social inclusion 154–6

Work Capability Assessment 46–8

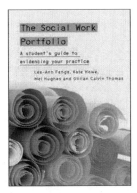

THE SOCIAL WORK PORTFOLIO
A STUDENT'S GUIDE TO EVIDENCING YOUR PRACTICE

Lee-Ann Fenge, Kate Howe, Mel Hughes and Gill Thomas

June 2014 114pp
978-0-335-24531-4 – Paperback

eBook also available

The portfolio is an essential part of the summative assessment within qualifying social work programmes. All students are required to complete a practice portfolio to provide evidence of their learning in practice. This essential book demonstrates how students can use the portfolio to demonstrate their learning in terms of developing core knowledge, values and skills.

Topics covered include:

- What a portfolio is, and how to make best use of it in your learning journey
- How to evidence your capability using the Professional Capabilities Framework for Social Workers
- How to reflect on your own learning needs and learning style
- How to work with your practice educator in terms of practice learning and portfolio development
- How to evidence the use of theory in your portfolio
- How to evidence meaningful service user and carer involvement within your placement and portfolio
- How to use your portfolio as a basis for future CPD learning, including the need to develop Personal Development Plans and the role of AYSE

Written by a team of experts from Bournemouth University, each chapter uses a range of reflective activities, practice educator comments, and student testimony to illustrate the discussion.

www.openup.co.uk

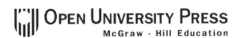

OPEN UNIVERSITY PRESS
McGraw - Hill Education

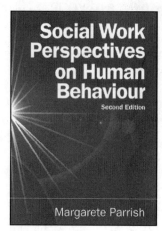

SOCIAL WORK PERSPECTIVES ON HUMAN BEHAVIOUR
Second Edition

Margarete Parrish

9780335262847 (Paperback)
9780335262854 (ebook)
2014

The capacity to observe, interpret and understand human behaviour is vital for effective social work practice. By choosing to enter a profession that requires high levels of astute observation and listening skills in the interpretation of people's behaviour, social work students have undertaken a demanding task.

Using a bio-psychosocial framework, this fascinating book provides a wide basis of perspectives on human behaviour on which to build understanding of and responses to people's behaviours, along with an enhanced appreciation of some of the circumstances that shape behaviour.

Key features:

- Exercises for students to complete
- Chapter summary points
- Discussion questions

www.openup.co.uk

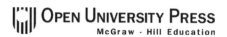 **OPEN UNIVERSITY PRESS**
McGraw · Hill Education